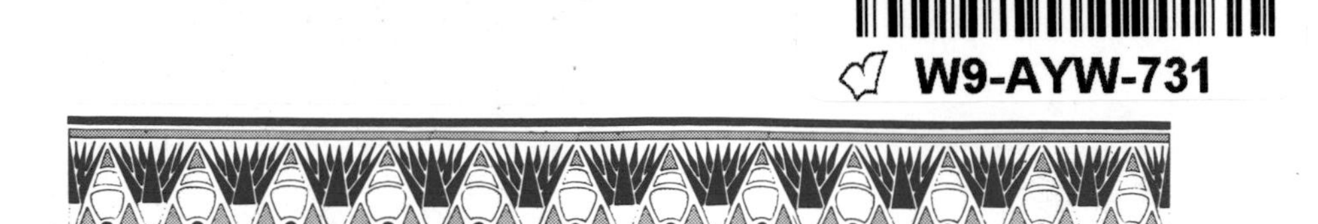

The Medical Skills of Ancient Egypt

J. WORTH ESTES

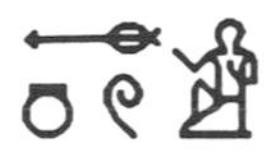

SCIENCE HISTORY PUBLICATIONS/U.S.A.
1989

If the publishers have unwittingly infringed
the copyright in any illustration reproduced,
they will gladly pay an appropriate fee
on being satisfied as to the owner's title.

First published in the United States of America
by Science History Publications/USA *a division of*
Watson Publishing International
Post Office Box 493
Canton, MA 02021

Library of Congress Cataloging-in-Publication Data

Estes, J. Worth, 1934–
The medical skills of ancient Egypt / J. Worth Estes.
p. cm.
Includes index.
ISBN 0-88135-093-1
1. Medicine, Egyptian. I. Title.
[DNLM: 1. History of Medicine, Ancient—Egypt. WZ 51 E79m]
R653.E4E87 1989
610'.932—dc19
DNLM/DLC
for Library of Congress 89-6004
CIP

Designed and manufactured in the U.S.A.

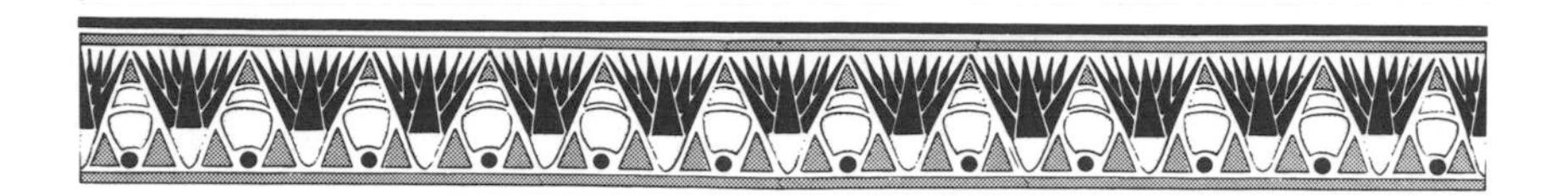

for SAMIHA BARKOUKY
who taught me about Egypt,

and PHILIP CASH
who is still teaching me about history

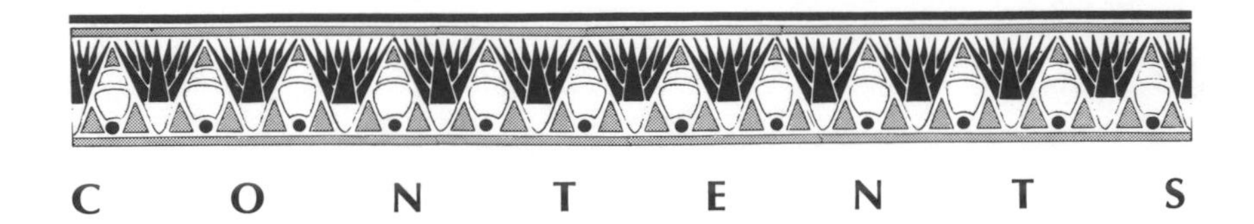

CONTENTS

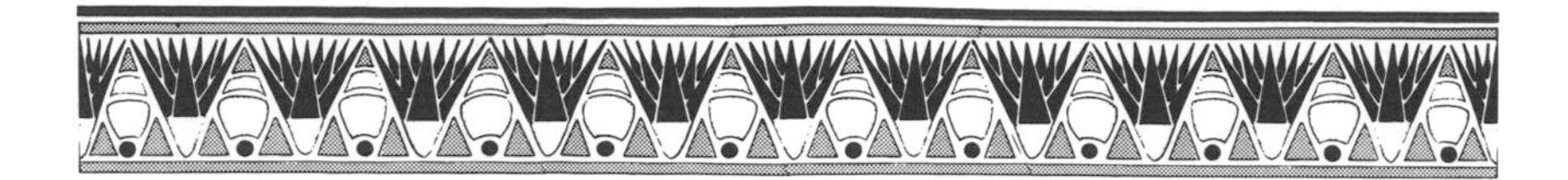

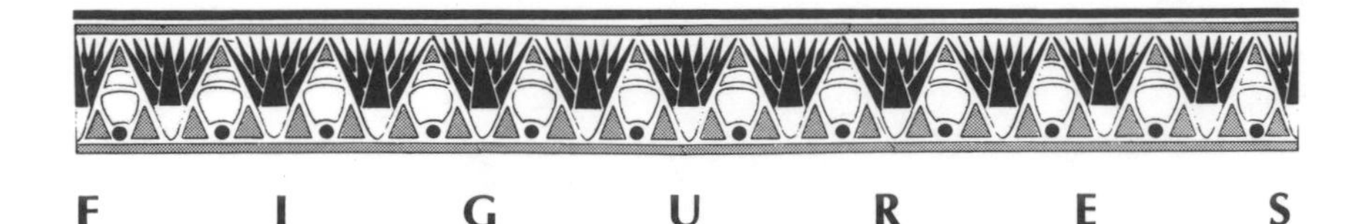

F I G U R E S

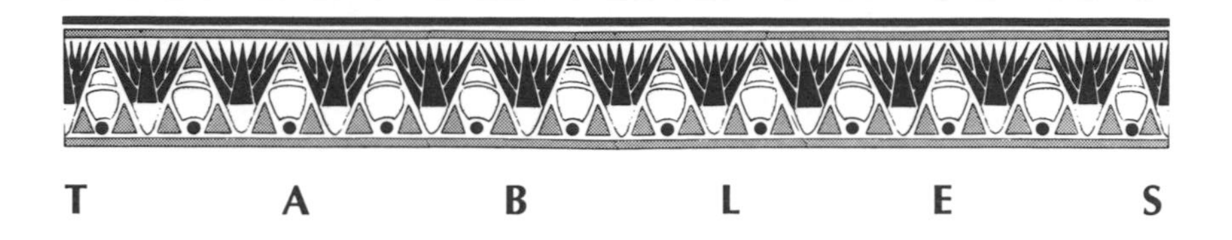

T A B L E S

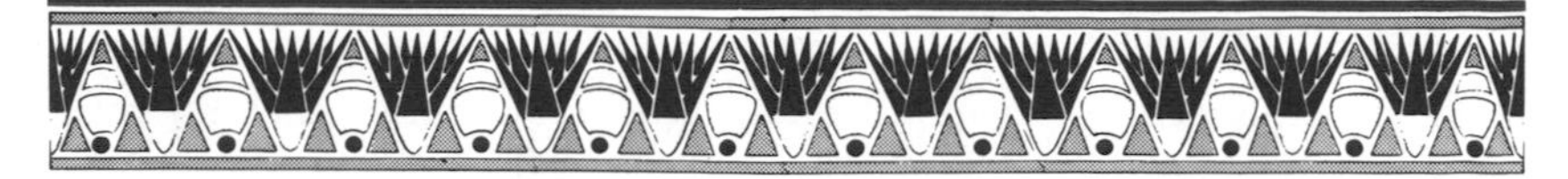

INTRODUCTION AND ACKNOWLEDGMENTS

This book began during a visit to Egypt in 1979. Because our extraordinary guide there, Samiha Barkouky, knew I was interested in the history of my profession, one day she brought along a lavishly illustrated French book on ancient Egyptian medicine for me to see. I read a chapter or two each night as we continued our travels because I was not optimistic that I could find a copy in the United States. However, to my great surprise, I found one in the gift shop of our hotel at Aswan several days later. When I settled down to read my prize more carefully at home, I began to think it might deserve an English translation.

But then I found that much new information had accumulated since the French book was written, and even more since the last works in English had appeared, so I began work on my own version of the story. A year or so later, I had to lay it aside in favor of projects with inescapable deadlines. By the time I could return to this one, six years had passed.

I have written this book for anyone who is interested in daily life in ancient Egypt, as well as for physicians who are interested in the development of their profession and for Egyptologists who are interested in health, disease, and medical treatments along the banks of the Nile. Most of my story takes place before the Greeks and Romans began to impose their own views and practices on the Egyptians, but I have not hesitated to use material from later centuries, especially when it reflects or illuminates older Egyptian practices.

It may not be not entirely appropriate to describe this book as a "story," since there is little evidence that ancient Egyptian medicine evolved or progressed in any way. I do not mean to imply that it was completely static, only that virtually no evidence of any changes that might have occurred has survived. Instead of telling a true story, then, I have tried to lay out a series—a collage, as it were—of snapshots that illustrate what can be inferred about Egyptians' illnesses and their treatments in the days of the pharaohs. In doing so, I have tried to avoid making (or confirming) conclusions or diagnoses that cannot be fully supported by the evidence available.

Some readers may be annoyed at my decision not to use footnote superscripts on every possible occasion. Instead, I have developed collective notes for the end of many paragraphs; the interested reader will be able to find all sources cited in the appropriate endnotes with minimal inconvenience.

Acknowledgments

Many people contributed in many ways to my understanding of ancient Egypt and its medical practices, beginning with Mrs. Barkouky— whose friendship my wife and I continue to enjoy and value. Those who have kindly sent me books, articles, and photocopies, or who have found elusive items for me, include: Richard J. Wolfe (Boston Medical Library), Dr. William F. McNary, Jr. (Boston University School of Medicine), Dr. John C. Kramer (University of California, Irvine), Dr. Eva B. Ryden (while a student at Tufts University School of Veterinary Medicine), Dr. LaVerne Kuhnke (Northeastern University), Dr. Eugene G. Laforet (Newton, Mass.), Dr. Bernadine Z. Paulshock (Wilmington, Del.), and Edward Pearce and Brent Jackson (both of the Boston Museum of Science). Dr. John Scarborough (then at the University of Kentucky) very kindly read and commented on my earliest drafts and supplied many new references and his own translation of a key passage in Herodotus. Ida Hay identified several plants used in Egyptian remedies with her customary skillful use of the vast library resources of the Arnold Arboretum, Boston.

Dr. Stanley Strzempko was an undergraduate at Colgate University in 1980–1981 when, in my laboratory, he learned a great deal about pharmacology by carrying out the experiments described in the Postscript to Chapter Three. Ellen O. Weinberg, a graduate student in pharmacology at Boston University, translated important articles from German for me. Among the Egyptologists who have sent me helpful materials and opinions are: Dr. Stuart Fleming (University of Pennsylvania), Dr. Robert S. Bianchi (The Brooklyn Museum), Dr. Alan R. Schulman (Queen's College of the City University of New York), and Dr. T. G. H. James (British Museum).

I am very grateful to Irene Buonopane for graciously contributing a drawing of the Step Pyramid at Sakkara, which she could base only on an assortment of diagrams and photographs I assembled for her. Fred Delorey (then of the Boston University School of Medicine Department of Educational Media) contributed a photograph of a modern sculpture of Imhotep.

Much of my research would not have been possible without the help I received from the staff of the Department of Egyptian and Ancient Near Eastern Art at the Museum of Fine Arts, Boston, and its library put almost all the literature of Egyptology at my fingertips. When I began my research, Dr. Susan K. Doll provided many valuable bibliographic clues. When I returned to it six years later, Dr. Edward Brovarski induced my wife and me to join the Friends of Egyptian Art, whose monthly meetings have provided valuable leads to pertinent current research. Many members of the department staff have found answers to my questions, and some, like Sue D'Auria, have shared their own research with me. In the latter respect, I am also especially grateful to Dr. Timothy Kendall (currently Acting Curator) for allowing me to use an interview he conducted with a modern folk healer, as well as for bibliographic suggestions and for permission to use photographs in his department's collection. I am also grateful to Dr. Cornelius Vermeule of the museum's Department of Classical Art for his hospitality in the library of his department.

But above all I am indebted to Yvonne J. Markowitz of the museum's Egyptian Department for many contributions that she very graciously volunteered. Not only did she (with Dr. Cynthia Rose of Brandeis University) translate a hieroglyphic text for me, she also made three skillful contour drawings and the lotus design for the chapter heads, and she composed the hieroglyphs, based chiefly on their usage in the definitive editions of the Smith and Ebers papyri, that are interspersed throughout my text. I can't thank her enough for all her efforts. In addition, Dr. Ann Roth of the same department kindly verified details in the drawing of the controversial tools carved on a wall at Kom Ombo while she was on a visit there.

Precisely because I am not an expert in Egyptology, I realized that someone who is should review my manuscript for errors that would shame a first-year student of the subject. Dr. Kathryn Bard (Department of Archaeology, Boston University) generously offered to take on that task. Not only did she correct a number of my errors, her comments also helped me to clarify some of my arguments. All my expressions of appreciation cannot be a sufficient reward to her.

But despite the help I've received, I must emphasize that any surviving errors of fact should be attributed only to me, not to any of my consultants, especially since I have felt free to disagree with a few of their views.

Finally, I am grateful to Joyce Becotte for her extraordinarily patient and skillful processing of my complicated and continually evolving manuscript. It was not an easy task.

J. W. E.

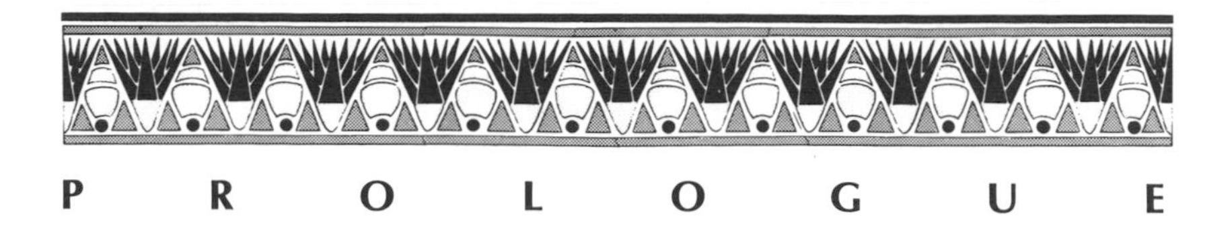

P R O L O G U E

IMHOTEP AND THE PYRAMIDS

Although Sir William Osler, a distinguished student of medicine's past, labelled an ancient Egyptian named Imhotep as "the first figure of a physician to stand out clearly from the mists of antiquity,"[1] there is absolutely no evidence that Imhotep ever practiced any of the healing arts. Nevertheless, by about 2000 years after his death, his countrymen had come to regard him as the preeminent healer in their history. How did Imhotep acquire his posthumous immortality, based on an unwarranted reputation that has persisted into our own time?

His story and its accompanying legends began during the first of the four flowerings of ancient Egyptian civilization, the one known today as the Old Kingdom (royal Dynasties III through VI, 2649–2150 B.C.). The Egyptians had had ox-drawn ploughs, potter's wheels, papyrus, boats with sails for water transport upstream, and domesticated asses for land transport for at least three centuries by then. They would not have vehicles with spoked wheels, much less wheeled transport, until ancient Egypt's third flowering as the New Kingdom (Dynasties XVIII to XX, 1550–1070 B.C.). Bronze was not widely used in the Nile valley until about six centuries after Imhotep died. A few iron implements had been imported as early as his lifetime, but the newer metal was never widely used in ancient Egypt.[2]

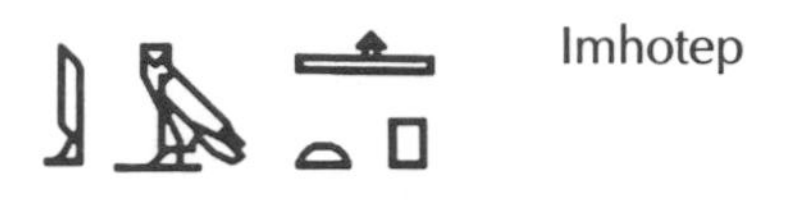

Imhotep

Imhotep was probably born around 2650 B.C. at Memphis, the capital city begun 300 years earlier by Narmer, the first king of the First Dynasty, after the unification of the even more ancient kingdoms of Upper and Lower Egypt. Imhotep's father, Kanofer, was said to have been a builder from whom the son learned the skills that would be necessary for his major accomplishment.[3]

Memphis was near modern Cairo, where the Upper Nile, its narrow valley still harshly bounded by the desert, empties into the lush alluvial delta of the Lower Nile. The arable extent of the kingdom was about 13,000 square miles, approximately the combined areas of Massachusetts and Connecticut. Today, more than 99.5 percent of the Egyptian population lives on this same 3.5 percent of the country's total area. The valley's fertility was renewed each summer by flood waters from highland Ethiopia and East Africa; rain is rare in Upper Egypt, and even in the delta where the Nile empties into the Mediterranean it amounts to no more than about eight inches a year.[4]

Imhotep's career probably began in one of the great temples of Memphis, perhaps one where the ibis-headed divine scribe Thoth was worshipped; his later work required detailed knowledge of the numbers, systems of measurement, and astronomical lore that Thoth, who was also a protector of the dead, was believed to have invented. According to

FIGURE 1. Map of ancient Egypt, showing sites mentioned throughout the text. Memphis became the capital of Old Kingdom Egypt because it was near the junction of the more ancient kingdoms of Lower and Upper Egypt. Thebes included Luxor and Karnak and is represented by the modern town of Luxor. The Nile was not navigable beyond the cataracts except by portage. The southern limit of ancient Egypt was at the first cataract of the Nile; the modern boundary between Egypt and the Sudan is between Abu Simbel and the second cataract. The star at the beginning of the Nile delta represents the modern capital, Cairo, which was settled after 969 A.D.

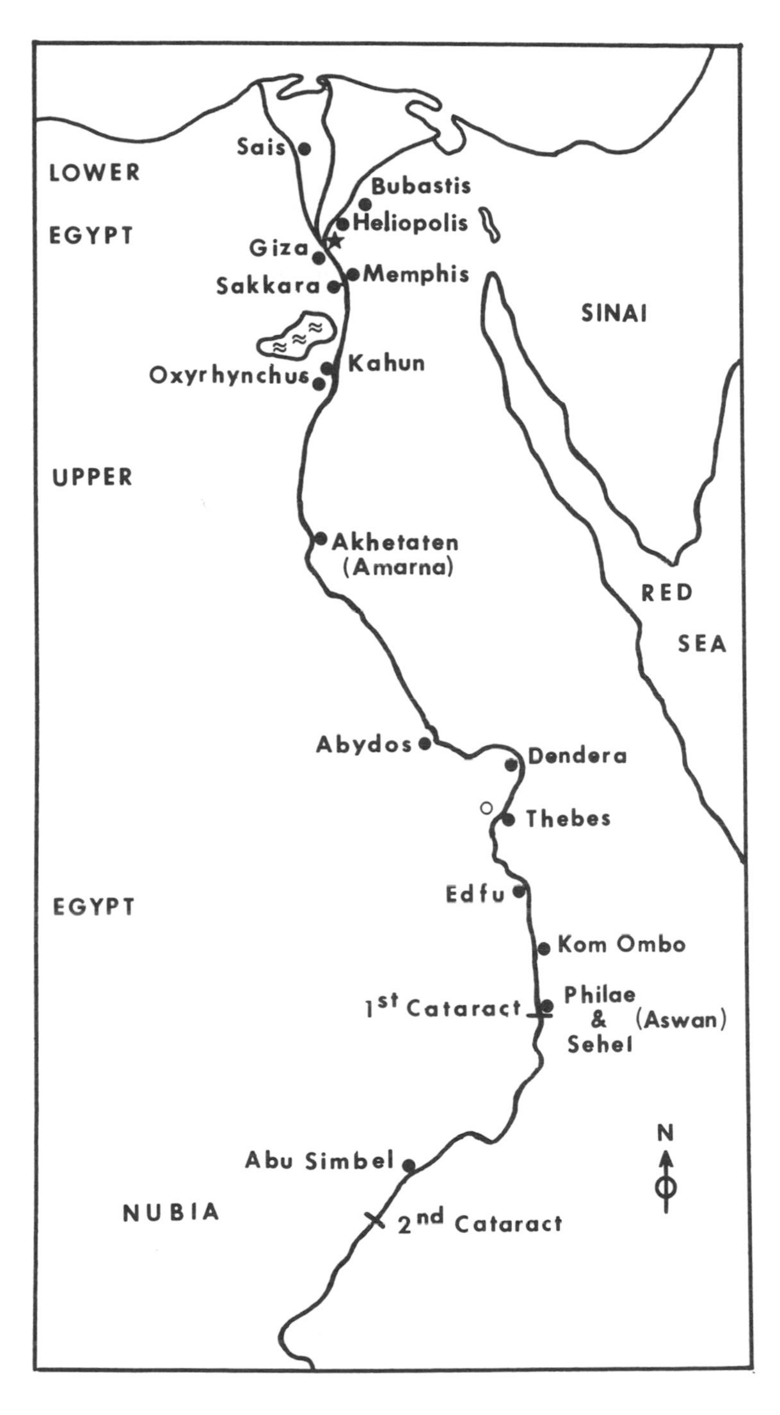

LOWER
EGYPT
UPPER
EGYPT
Sais
Bubastis
Heliopolis
Giza
Memphis
Sakkara
SINAI
Kahun
Oxyrhynchus
Akhetaten
(Amarna)
RED
SEA
Abydos
Dendera
Thebes
Edfu
Kom Ombo
1st Cataract
Philae
&
Sehel
(Aswan)
N
Abu Simbel
NUBIA
2nd Cataract

later traditions, Imhotep wrote about architecture and medicine (another of Thoth's associations), among other subjects, but none of his writings has survived. Even so, a poet of the twentieth century B.C. used Imhotep's books to exemplify ideals of wisdom that had outlasted their author's monuments in stone. In a song from the Middle Kingdom (Dynasty XI, 2040–1991 B.C.), Imhotep's architectural inventions, and those of Cheops' son Hardedef, symbolize the futility of earthly grandeur, and are contrasted with the far longer survival of their written wisdom:

The gods who were before rest in their tombs.
Blessed nobles too are buried in their tombs.
(Yet) those who built tombs,
Their places are gone,
What has become of them?
I have heard the words of Imhotep and Hardedef,
Whose sayings are recited whole.
What of their places?
Their walls have crumbled,
Their places are gone,
As though they had never been!
None comes from there,
To tell of their state,
To tell of their needs,
To calm our hearts,
Until we go where they have gone![5]

Eventually Imhotep became chief priest of the sun god Rē at the ancient cult center at Heliopolis, 25 miles north of Memphis. His accompanying title "Chief of the Observers" suggests that he took the sky-watching skills he had learned as a priest of Thoth to his new position. As chief priest he would have supervised the rituals surrounding the statue of the god who made his home in the temple. This meant that Imhotep probably began his day by sprinkling the statue with water, clothing and anointing it, applying cosmetic pigments to its golden eyes, presenting food offerings, and then reciting appropriate prayers as the idol was carried into the sunlit courtyard. Similarly, the priest's day would have ended by reversing this ritual, when the statue was put to rest in the temple's innermost sanctuary for the night. Imhotep might also have officiated at interments at the nearby necropolis, when life was ritually restored to the mummified body just before it was laid into its tomb.[6]

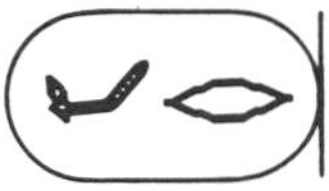

Zoser

At about this time the pharaoh Zoser (2630–2611 B.C.), son of the founder of the Third Dynasty and of the Old Kingdom, came to the throne. He moved his court from the ancient cult center at Abydos, in Upper Egypt, to Memphis. Ruling for nearly 20 years, Zoser (also transliterated as Djoser) seems to have completed the consolidation of Upper and Lower Egypt. The head of an increasingly powerful central government, in which he functioned as both religious and secular head, Zoser delegated much of his authority to bureaucrats. Among these functionaries Imhotep took a leading role, eventually becoming the king's vizier, or chancellor. Still chief priest of Rē in all Egypt, Imhotep as Zoser's principal executive officer came to be the apex of a vast bureaucracy reporting directly to the king.[7]

The word "Imhotep" means something like "he who comes in peace," or "he who satisfies," depending on how idiomatically one reads hieroglyphs. The phrase was in common use in ancient Egypt. For instance, in the "Book of the Dead" as preserved in the much later Papyrus of Ani, the deceased prays that his body not be separated from his soul at the gates of the underworld, and that Ani be allowed to enter and leave the netherworld "in peace," which is written with the same hieroglyphs that were used in Imhotep's name.[8] Clearly, Zoser was satisfied with his vizier.

His most solid and lasting achievement still rises out of the desert overlooking the meager ruins of Memphis on the west bank of the Nile: the Step Pyramid at Sakkara, which was the necropolis for the capital city. The tomb of Imhotep's king occupies a special place in the history of civilization: not only was it the first pyramid built in Egypt, it is also the oldest—and probably the first—large-scale stone building in the world.

Until Imhotep invented the monumental pyramid tomb, most Egyptian noblemen and royalty were buried in, or under, rectangular mounds of mud brick that archaeologists call mastabas (from the Arabic word for the stone bench that they resemble). People of lesser means (everyone, for that matter, in Predynastic Egypt, before about 3000 B.C.) were buried in simple grave pits, and were as well supplied for their journies through the next world as their circumstances would allow. Throughout their long history, the ancient Egyptians' burial practices reflected their belief that even after death men lived much as they had before.

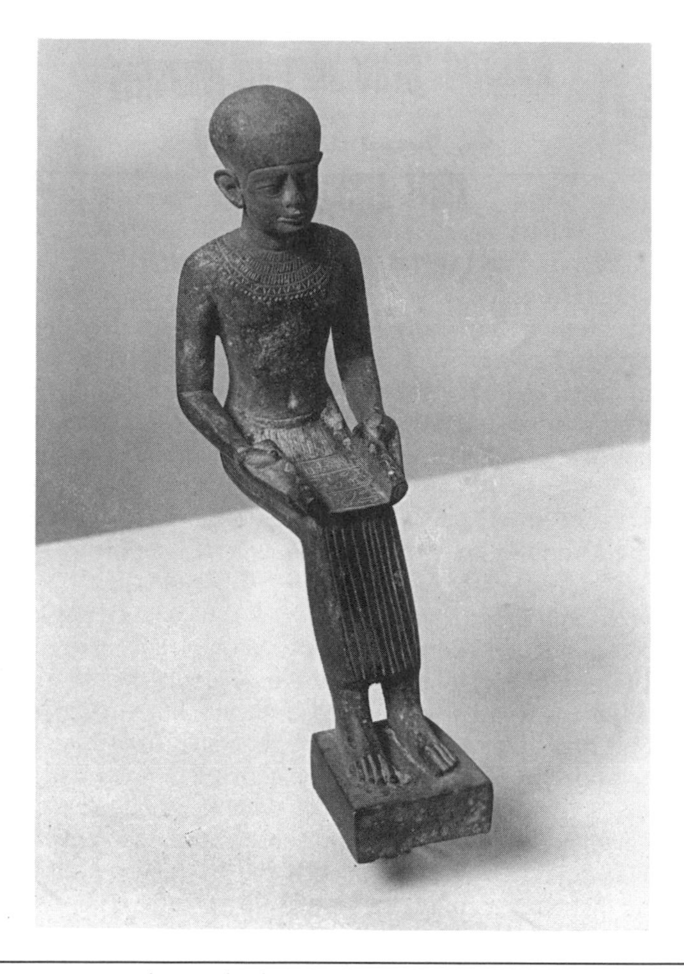

FIGURE 2. Bronze figure of Imhotep, 19 centimeters high, made between about 685 and 31 B.C. and excavated at Giza. The inscription on the scroll in his lap reads "Imhotep, the great one, son of Ptah, born of Kherednankh." (Courtesy, Museum of Fine Arts, Boston, 27.984)

Although the Egyptians believed that a man had three kinds of soul, several of their funeral practices focussed on the one called the *ka*. "That detached part of the personality which planned and acted for the rest of the person," the *ka* was a vital force which possessed all the characteristics of the deceased; it existed independently of him; and it enjoyed life with the gods in heaven when it wished. Thus, as an identical twin, it accompanied a person "through life as the sustaining constructing force, and preceded him in death to effect his successful existence in the next world."[9] Because of the *ka*'s overriding importance, those who had sufficient resources endowed *ka*-priests who were charged to provide food and other offerings, at the time of burial and in perpetuity, for the *ka* whose post-mortem dwelling places were the mummy and statues of the deceased.

Several architectural precedents for Imhotep's monumental invention have been hypothesized. Until recently it was generally surmised that he began in the traditional manner by building a large mastaba for his king over a 23-foot-square pit hollowed 92 feet down into the bedrock of the plateau at Sakkara to receive Zoser's sarcophagus. Then, to further magnify his sovereign's power, Imhotep was assumed simply to have enlarged the mastaba's dimensions by adding three more graduated layers above it, followed by two even higher steps; these additions necessitated further enlargement of the base, the original mastaba, until it covered about 3.5 acres. In the end, the completed tomb rose 204 feet above the low desert on the west bank of the Nile,[10] as seen in Figure 3.

But Imhotep was probably inspired by other prototypes as well. The Step Pyramid's only surviving precedent in the same vast necropolis is a rectangular tomb (no. 3038) built over a large burial pit during the First Dynasty (2920–2770 B.C.) reign of Adjib. On three sides the mudbrick memorial rises in eight easily climbable steps to a platform that was originally surmounted by a mastaba-like superstructure decorated to resemble a palace facade; the fourth side was smooth, without steps.[11] Other possible models for Imhotep's innovation have emerged from recent excavations in the royal necropolis that was begun at Abydos about

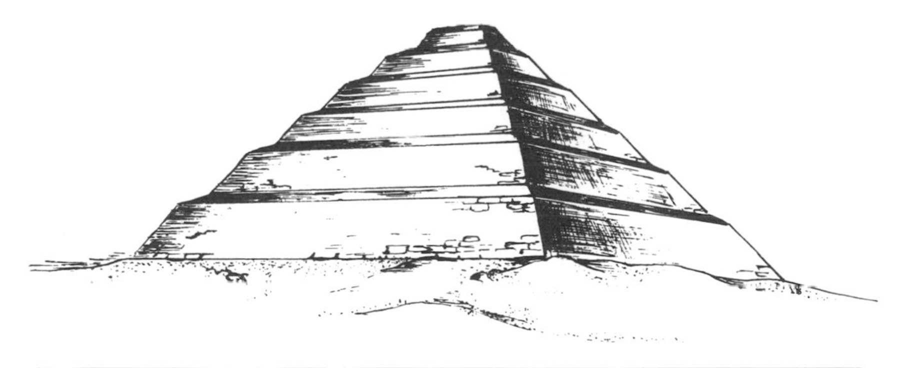

FIGURE 3. The Step Pyramid at Sakkara. Drawing by Irene Buonopane.

350 years before one was started at Sakkara. Several First Dynasty tombs at Abydos consisted of underground chambers covered by stepped cubes or rectangles made of brick and measuring 30 to 70 feet on a side. These graduated brick roofs could not have been visible once the tombs had been completed because they were enclosed by brick walls, also decorated like palaces, and then completely covered with sand and gravel.[12]

Around his Step Pyramid, Imhotep built a stone wall about 33 feet high and a little over a mile in circumference to enclose the 37 acres of ceremonial courts and buildings designed for the use of the king's *ka* and the priests of his funerary cult. The only architectural precedents for this part of his pioneering building project in quarried stone had been made of mud brick, wood, reeds, and other organic materials. Consequently, Imhotep's decorative inspirations recapitulated those traditional architectural forms in many details. For instance, the stones over the entrance passage were rounded to resemble palm logs, and the ritual temples in the courtyard had slightly curved roofs like those of buildings roofed with reeds.[13] The outside wall surface closely resembled the palace wall facades of many mastabas at Sakkara and Abydos. In addition, Abydos boasts the largest free-standing mud brick monument in the world, the 2.5-acre burial enclosure called the Shunet el Zebib. The niches in that 36-foot-high wall may have provided additional inspiration for the enclosure wall at Sakkara, built about 50 years later.[14]

Another of Imhotep's structural innovations was the stone column, although none of his was free standing. Because his principal building material was a relatively soft limestone, he joined his columns in pairs connected by walls of solid stone blocks, or attached them to walls for decorative purposes. He decorated his columns to resemble traditional wooden corner posts or bundles of reeds, and their capitals to represent what were then familiar plant and flower forms. Although Imhotep may have been unsure of a stone column's ability to support great weights, he seems to have been quite sure of his king's mastery over Egypt. The priest-architect gave the royal funerary complex a previously unknown grandeur, displaying Zoser's unchallenged power for all to see.[15]

To house the traditional statue in which the king's *ka* resided, Imhotep built a small stone edifice now called a *serdab* at the base of the pyramid. From two small holes facing north, Zoser's seated statue could view the universe, as well as the religious rituals in his honor, and through those holes his *ka*-spirit would be able to recognize its home, the awe-inspiring statue of the king[16] that is one of the truly great sculptures in history.

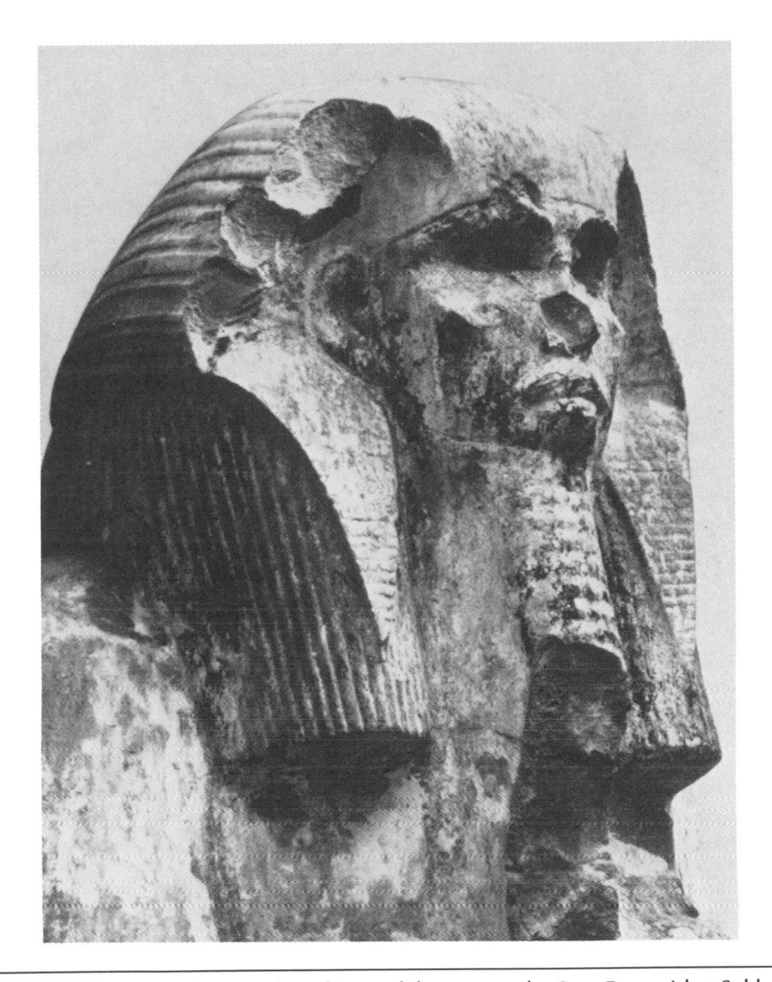

FIGURE 4. Head of Zoser, from his *serdab* statue at the Step Pyramid at Sakkara. The statue is in the Museum of Egyptian Antiquities, Cairo, and a reproductlon has been installed in the *serdab*. (Photograph in collection of the author.)

The Step Pyramid at Sakkara was the first in a series of experiments that culminated at nearby Giza a century later in the Great Pyramid of Cheops (2551–2528 B.C.; the Greeks and later generations called him Cheops, but his contemporaries knew him as Khufu or Khufwey). More pyramids were built over the next seven centuries, although their size gradually diminished as later kings came to realize that even these massive constructions could not protect their gold-laden mummies and luxurious funerary equipment from tomb robbers. Beginning in Dynasty XVIII (1550–1307 B.C.), royal tombs were carved into the Theban cliffs on the west bank of the Nile opposite modern Luxor. About 80 pyramids still stand along the Nile; none of these "most massive facts of antiquity"[17] has escaped the tomb robbers. But the relative sizes and construction techniques of the surviving pyramids still reflect their owners' respective abilities to marshal manpower and resources, capacities that reached extraordinary peaks under both Zoser and Cheops.[18]

Although the evidence is good that the first pyramid was indeed designed and built by Imhotep, and that he may have designed another (although it was never finished) for Zoser's successor, Sekhemkhet (2611–2603 B.C.), we do not know why he chose this form of funerary monument for Zoser. Perhaps he merely perpetuated and expanded forms used earlier at Sakkara and Abydos, but the continuing popularity of burial pyramids was probably associated with the development of additional religious implications. One school of thought suggests that pyramids came to represent the primeval earth mound on which the first god was made manifest. Another, that does not necessarily exclude the first, suggests that the steps of Imhotep's pyramid represent a staircase on which the king's spirit, or spirits, could climb to heaven, and that the true smooth-sided pyramids such as those at Giza, which were much more difficult to construct, represent the sun's rays on which the king, as the sun god's most exalted priest, could accomplish the same journey after death.[19]

Whatever Imhotep was trying to accomplish, he succeeded in devising an awesome symbol of the authority of a powerful monarch who had consolidated his kingdom's resources and provinces from the Mediterranean to Aswan. The Step Pyramid certainly set an appropriately grand precedent for succeeding Old Kingdom royal tomb complexes, which came to include a temple on the river front for receiving and preparing the body, a ceremonial causeway leading up toward the pyramid, and, at the base of the pyramid, a temple in which the posthumously deified king was worshipped, and where the supplies he would need in the afterlife were stored. Unfortunately, we can never know exactly what went on in Imhotep's mind as he chose the architectural design that became Egypt's "trademark" throughout the world—his chief purpose, after all, was simply to aggrandize his king.

There is little doubt that Zoser's vizier and chief priest deserves to be remembered today for inventing the pyramid. But, paradoxically, this quintessential professional bureaucrat is now more often remembered, despite the absence of corroborative evidence, as a physician, a role for which there is no documentary evidence from Dynasty III. In 1928 he appeared on an Egyptian postage stamp commemorating both the centennial of the medical school at Cairo and an international history of medicine meeting. Modern versions of his likeness appear on the facade of the Joslin Clinic in Boston and in the lobby of the Boston University School of Medicine, while that school and others have published senior class yearbooks titled *The Imhotepian*. Why?

Before we try to answer that question, we will review what is known about medical practice in ancient Egypt, up to the time when Greek and Roman medical practices and cultures replaced those of pharaonic civilization. Along the way we will examine the work of known Egyptian healers, including their surgical techniques and their drug remedies, as well as their patients and their patients' illnesses. Then, finally, we will return to the question of Imhotep, to discover why he is not the hero of this book, even if his legend has provided its theme.

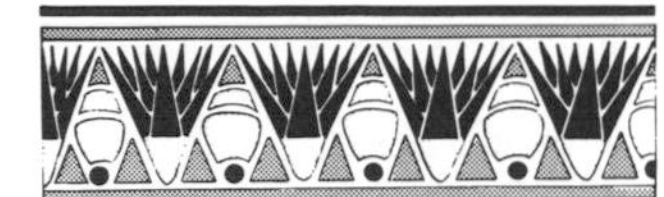

1

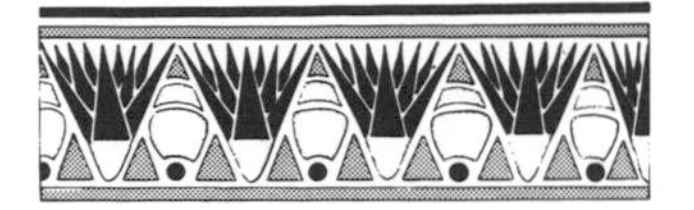

EGYPTIAN HEALERS

The few medical papyri that have survived since pharaohs ruled along the banks of the Nile form a fairly representative sampling of the world's first body of specifically medical literature, even if we cannot know the extent to which those works were actually read or consulted by ancient healers. The true origins of their skills remain obscure, but they almost certainly lie within the Egyptians' beliefs about the supernatural[1] (with the possible exception of the more pragmatic problem-solving approaches used in ancient surgery).

"Religion" and beliefs about "the supernatural" were probably not equal contributors to the development of the ancient Egyptians' medical practices. Since the primary purpose of their organized religion was to serve and justify the state, it is difficult to agree with Morenz that, "Religion was the basis of Egyptian medicine. Death was seen as caused by a message from the deity, except in those cases where violence was obviously involved," or that "the religious origin of art and science is fundamental [to Egyptian studies] as is the case in all other cultures as well."[2]

The concept of "science" implicit in such statements differs significantly from that used in modern medicine or other laboratory-based disciplines. When we talk of the "scientific method" today, we mean the process by which planned or chance observations give rise to hypotheses that are then tested experimentally (usually with appropriate controls) in such a way that they can then be accepted or rejected, and the results may even generate new hypotheses for further experimental testing. By contrast, statements about Egyptian "science" such as the one cited above really refer to the development of the *content*—the facts—that finally found a place in modern scientific vocabularies. Thus, just as astronomy almost certainly began with the need to understand celestial regularities for ritual purposes and for making agricultural predictions, so did medicine arise from attempts to interpret the symptoms of illness; it is likely that, in the beginning, supernatural interpretations furnished all the explanation that was necessary. Ancient Egyptians did not employ anything like today's scientific method in either astronomy or medicine, even if they did recognize astronomical and pathological phenomena that are still accepted facts. Disease and its symptoms were far more likely to be ascribed to local, or minor, supernatural influences than to malevolent forces emanating from the great gods of the state. Indeed, these gods seem to have been fairly benevolent on the whole.

Death was a constant threat to ancient Egyptians, and while they feared it, they were not depressed or pessimistic about it because they believed in a life after death, even if they were not complacent about the next world.[3] Spells and incantations were often used in the treatment of illness, which was probably regarded as one step on the way toward eventual death. Most of the surviving medico-magical spells were written down during the later centuries of Egyptian history and even into the Christian era, but they probably preserve ideas that had first emerged many centuries earlier.

The Chester Beatty V Papyrus, which dates from Dynasty XIX (1307–1196 B.C.), the family of Ramesses II, contains typical spells. One for exorcising a headache begins by asking 20 gods "to remove that enemy, dead man or dead woman, adversary male or female which is the face of N [the patient's name], born of M." The healer is then told to recite the spell "over a crocodile of clay with grain in its mouth, and its eye of faience set [in] its head. One shall tie [?] [it] and inscribe a drawing of the gods upon a strip of fine linen to be placed upon his head." Finally, the spell is to be recited over images of 11 gods "and an oryx on whose back stands a figure [probably of the god Horus] carrying his lance." The next incantation treats the headache as if it were a demon by threatening to burn its soul and consume its corpse, followed by a litany of further threats that the healer will employ if the headache does not succumb to the first.[4]

A propagandistic inscription found at Karnak and purporting to be from the same period, although it was actually written some 900 years later, recounts the story of Bentresh, the sister of a Hittite princess who had become one of the queens of Ramesses II. When Bentresh became ill, Ramesses was asked to send a learned man, a healer, to the Hittite court. He "found Bentresh to be possessed by a spirit . . . an enemy against whom one could not fight." In desperation the Egyptian envoy wrote home to ask his king to send a god to cure the princess. Ramesses then consulted a local deity, Khons-in-Thebes-Neferhotep, and he, in turn, sent one of his own lesser manifestations who also possessed healing skills, Khons-the-Provider, "the great god who expels disease demons." When he arrived at the court of Bentresh's father in Bakhtan, in what is now Turkey, the god cast a spell and the girl became well.[5]

The so-called Leiden Papyrus is a collection of spells for a wide range of purposes (not all of them for healing) written down in the third century A.D. Some were probably no more than 100 or 200 years old by then, although a few may date from as early as the New Kingdom. The papyrus provides incantations for problems such as "extracting the venom from the heart of a man who has been made to drink a potion," one to be "spoken to [a] man, when a bone has stuck in his throat," and a talisman for the foot of a man with "gout." Another spell was to be "spoken to the bite of the dog," although it concludes with the suggestion that the wound be cleaned and treated first with salt and then dressed with an ointment of honey; as will be seen later, honey was a conventional wound remedy that was likely to have speeded normal wound healing.[6]

Other spells in the same papyrus are designed to cause illness. For instance, to blind a man, put a powdered mouse in his drink, or, to kill him, put the ground mouse in his food; after he eats it, he will swell up and die. Another recipe tells how the same mouse can be used as an aphrodisiac. Scattered throughout the papyrus are recipes for ointments composed of ingredients such as crocodile and antelope dungs, ass placenta, male goat gall, foam from a stallion's mouth, acacia pods, honey, alum, pepper, and assorted unidentified plant materials, which a woman can put on her husband's phallus, so that he will make love to her. And finally, among a number of drug remedies that will be discussed later are some that reflect a mixture of magic and pharmacological effect, such as recipes that will make a man sleep. Some of these include ingredients that have been translated as opium, hyoscyamus, and mandragora; if those translations are accurate—and they probably are not (see the Appendix)—such drugs might indeed have done what was intended.[7]

Even in papyri that are clearly more "medical" than "magical," we find spells which will assist the healer or his drugs. One of the most famous, the Ebers Papyrus (see Chapter Four), begins with a spell to be recited when applying a remedy to an arm or leg:

> *I have come from Heliopolis with the old ones in the temple, the possessors of protection, the rulers of eternity; assuredly, I have come from Sais with the mother of the gods. They have given me their protection. I have formulas composed by the lord of the universe in order to expel afflictions [caused] by a god or goddess, by dead man or woman, etc.*[8]

Another spell in the same document is to be recited when drinking a remedy:

> *Come remedy! Come thou who expellest [evil] things in this my stomach and in these my limbs! . . . Dost thou remember that [the gods] Horus and Seth have been conducted to the big palace at Heliopolis, when there was negotiated of Seth's testicles with Horus, and he shall get well like one who is on earth. He does all that he may wish like these gods who are there.*

The writer of this spell added that it is very powerful, especially when repeated backward.[9]

Magical objects were used in Egyptian healing as well as spoken spells. Amulets warded off disease-producing demons, while talismans acted as personal vehicles for carrying beneficent forces created by magical rites. Some of each were carved, while others were written on papyrus; when the latter were soaked in water, the ink would run off, transferring the magic to anyone who drank the water or washed an appropriate part of his body with it.[10]

The same function was also served by healing statues. Many showed the god Horus as a child, standing on a crocodile, while others represented men holding miniature versions of similar statues. Horus was invoked especially for the treatment of snakebites, a common hazard of daily life in ancient Egypt. As a boy, he had survived a snakebite with the help of the god Thoth, who made him immune to snakes thereafter. Surviving examples of both statue types were designed to impregnate water flowing over them with sufficient power to heal a patient who had been bitten by a snake when he drank or bathed in the water.[11]

The ancient Egyptians had no god devoted only to medicine until late in their history. Instead, healing roles were assigned to several gods in the pantheon, as minor correlates to their myths, during the 3000 years before a single god was appointed to that task. For instance, Isis became associated with healing because, in the great national myth, she had put the dismembered body of her husband Osiris back together (after which he impregnated her with Horus).

Egyptian temples were designed not for congregational worship but as settings in which the priests carried out their rituals. However, some temples were also associated with healing. At those temples, the transference of magical healing powers via water was practiced on a large scale in buildings now called sanitoria, such as that at the temple of Hathor at Dendera. Although its present buildings were erected during the Ptolemaic and Roman periods, they reflect practices that had probably originated many centuries earlier. The sick could bathe in water that had been sanctified, perhaps in the temple's sacred lake, so that they would be healed by being imbued with the same vital forces that had regenerated Osiris after Isis had restored his body. Another curative procedure used at Dendera and elsewhere in the Late Period (712–332 B.C.) was incubation, which required the sick person to spend a night in the sanitorium with the expectation that the god would cause him to dream his cure.[12]

Since magical spells and invocations to the gods could produce desirable outcomes like the prevention or cure of illness, we are not surprised that two of the three best-defined classes of ancient Egyptian healers were magicians and priests. People who functioned only as magicians, however, are not very prominent in the surviving records, possibly because they were few in number, and because magical methods for dealing with the supernatural—such as spells and incantations—were also important facets of the work of the two more prominent classes of healers, certain priest-physicians and the lay physicians called *swnw*[13] (probably pronounced something like *sounou*).

The professional medical training of the priest-physicians was probably the same as that of the lay physicians. Both examined their patients and then treated them with spells and drugs. Most visible among the religious practitioners were the priests of the lion-headed goddess Sekhmet, who could inflict plagues, war, and death. However, not all of her priests were healers; many were administrators or experts on ritual practices. "Lector-priests" comprised a second group of clerical healers, although they were more concerned with temple and funeral rituals. Somewhat inferior in status, they may have acquired anatomical knowledge pertinent to some aspects of healing in the embalming room, although that seems doubtful. Last among the priestly healers were those who provided food and other supplies for the *ka* spirits who resided in the necropolis to which the priests were attached; they also performed ritual circumcisions (see Chapter Three).[14]

Swnw

Although the title *swnw* was given to many healing priests, most of the known *swnw* were lay physicians; some were also scribes (*sš swnw*, pronounced *sesh sounou*). Their sources of medical training are completely unknown. Although professional knowledge may well have been transmitted from father to son,[15] only one family in which that occurred (over three generations) can be documented.[16] Some *swnw* may have received on-the-job training as apprentices, perhaps under the auspices of temples, but no definite evidence for such arrangements has surfaced. The two lowest ranks in the medical scale were the bandagers, a job that probably grew out of the embalming procedure, and an ill-defined group of trainees; both were supervised by physicians.[17]

Swnw probably learned little or nothing of medical value from the mummification process, partly because anatomic investigations were not, or could not be, carried out on cadavers for both climatic and religious reasons, and partly because the embalmers' lower place in society precluded their participation in "scholarly activities" alongside the more learned professions. Although the Egyptians gave names to many parts of the body, most of those were externally visible or prominent within the body cavities, so their mere indentification was not very academically "anatomical." However, there is evidence that physicians did perform autopsies in Greco-Roman Egypt.[18] Although the heart and the vessels that connected it with other body parts were described in several medical papyri, those descriptions were based more on speculation than on observation, as we will see.

One institution associated with temples may, arguably, have been closely concerned with medicine: the House of Life (*per ankh*). At least five are known. They were attached to temples at Bubastis and Sais in the delta, and at Abydos, Edfu, and the short-lived capital city Akhetaten at the site now called Tell el-Amarna, all in Upper Egypt. No lay *swnw* seems to have been associated with any of them, although a New Kingdom *swnw* rebuilt the House of Life at the temple of Neith at Abydos. Many centuries later an Egyptian naval officer named Udjahorresne (or Udjahorresnet) became a leading courtier and chief physician to Cambyses after the Persian king conquered Egypt in 525 B.C. Cambyses' successor, Darius I (ruled Egypt 521–486 B.C.), sent Udjahorresne to revive the House of Life at Sais because it had fallen on bad times. An inscription on Udjahorresne's statue, which is now in the Vatican, specifies that one good reason for restoring the Sais *per ankh* was that its staff "make live all that are sick." These still only vaguely defined institutions seem to have functioned much like medieval European monastic scriptoria, or collegial centers of learning. By the Late Period, books on medicine as well as on magic, theology, ritual, dream interpretation, and temple administration were being copied out and consulted in the Houses of Life. Thus, the medical papyri may have been written in *per ankh*s and used by *swnw* who went there to consult the texts, but none of these institutions seems to have functioned in any way as a medical school.[19] The great Museum at Alexandria, founded about 295 B.C. during the early Ptolemaic period, shared many roles, including medical ones, with the Houses of Life. Indeed, the Museum may have been closely modelled on those Egyptian institutions, although unequivocal evidence is lacking.[20]

Paul Ghalioungui has catalogued 54 documented Old Kingdom healers, 20 from the Middle Kingdom, 40 from the New Kingdom, and 15 from the Late Period, as well as 26 more for whom the documentation is less convincing. Two-thirds (86) of the 129 known healers were clearly labelled as *swnw*; some were also magicians or priests, while a variety of titles was applied to the rest. During the Old Kingdom, *swnw* held positions such as Chief, Inspector, Overseer, or Master of Physicians, and Chief of Physicians of the North (i.e., Lower Egypt) or the South (Upper Egypt), but the only titles that seem to have survived into later eras were the *swnw* and the Chief of Physicians (*wr swnw*, pronounced something like *oor sounou*). Despite the elaborate titulary, however, nothing is known of their hierarchical organization or of their professional subordinates at court or elsewhere.[21]

Some *swnw* had additional titles suggesting that they specialized in the various parts of the body: Physician of the Eyes, Physician of the

Belly, Shepherd of the Anus, and Chief of Dentists.[22] In about 425 B.C. the Greek historian Herodotus wrote of the Egyptians:

> *The practice of medicine they split into separate parts, each doctor being responsible for the treatment of only one disease. There are, in consequence, innumerable doctors, some specializing in diseases of the eye, others of the head, others of the stomach, and so on; while others, again, deal with the sort of troubles which cannot be exactly localized.*[23]

Some *swnw* may well have earned special reputations in treating inflammation around the eye, since several of their ointments probably did have effective antimicrobial properties (see Chapter Three). However, specialization by internal organs would seem to have been unlikely in ancient Egyptian medical thought and practice, since, as will be seen, the *swnw* assumed that almost all illnesses arose from a single underlying cause. The usual translation "Shepherd of the Anus" should probably be altered to reflect the fact that the word commonly translated as "anus" really refers to the entire lower gastrointestinal tract below the stomach. Thus, it seems likely that the area of major medical interest to the "Shepherd of the Anus" really coincided with that of the "Physician of the Belly." Alternatively, the "Shepherd of the Anus" may have been only a royal enema-maker.[24]

Herodotus' description of the *swnw* raises other issues as well. It is possible that Herodotus was being less complimentary to Egyptian physicians than might be inferred from the translation given above. John Scarborough translates the same passage as:

> *Medicine is thereby divided among [the Egyptians] so that each doctor knows but one disease and none of the others. All [Egypt] is stuffed with physicians: some appoint [themselves as experts] on eyes, others "do" the head, others teeth, others matters having to do with the belly, and others "specialize" in hidden diseases.*

This interpretation implies that an ancient Egyptian knew that someone was a doctor because he *said* he was; Herodotus' use of the word "stuffed" (in Greek, *plea*) suggests to Scarborough that the ancient historian saw, or presumed, a great deal of quackery,[25] at least by the standards of Classical Greece. An altogether different problem is raised by the probability that Herodotus did not himself visit Egypt,[26] which makes it even more difficult to accept his description of "specialization," although a few other texts[27] do seem to confirm it, at least for earlier periods.

The extent to which any *swnw* practiced dentistry is also problematic. The few remedies for ailments of the teeth and gums given in the Ebers Papyrus may have assuaged at least some of the many victims of caries and severely worn teeth, but there is little evidence of operative dental work in any of the mummies that have been studied. Such negative evidence must be weighed against descriptions of four or five *swnw*, and two men who were not *swnw*, as dentists (literally, "toothists") or otherwise concerned with the teeth. Inscriptions in the mastaba of Hesy-Rē (see Figure 5) at Sakkara describe him as Chief Physician, Chief Dentist, Royal Scribe, Chief Architect, High Priest of the Sanctuary of Min (the perpetually erect fertility god), Chief of the Ten of the South, and Dean of the Service of Offerings. Because he probably served Zoser (and therefore may have known Imhotep), his portrayals on several wooden panels in his mastaba appear to be the oldest known pictures of any *swnw*, or of any dentist.[28]

Perhaps the most surprising among the known *swnw* is a woman named Peseshet who lived during the Old Kingdom. She was Lady Overseer of Lady Physicians (*swnw.t*, probably pronounced *sounou et*), which implies that other women were practicing medicine with her.[29] The only other woman among the known physicians of ancient Egypt, named Tawe, was mentioned in an early Ptolemaic papyrus.[30]

Most physicians seem to have been held in high esteem in ancient Egypt, although their position probably owed as much to their association with learning and books as to their roles as healers. When Wesh-Ptah, the vizier and Chief Architect of the Dynasty V pharaoh Neferirkare (2446–2426 B.C.), fell down sick during a royal inspection tour of a new building project, the king himself tried to raise him from the ground:

> *But Wesh-Ptah remained prostrate and Pharaoh, the royal children, and the court were greatly scared. Then the king had Wesh-Ptah carried to the palace, and summoned the royal children, the lector priests and the physicians. The books were brought and consulted. But the verdict [prognosis] was hopeless and Pharaoh, full of sorrow, repaired to his apartments to pray to Rē daily for the life of his beloved vizier.*[31]

Not only does this story illustrate the association of physicans and lector-priests as well as reliance on medical texts for treating the sick, it also demonstrates that such documents were available as early as Dynasty V.

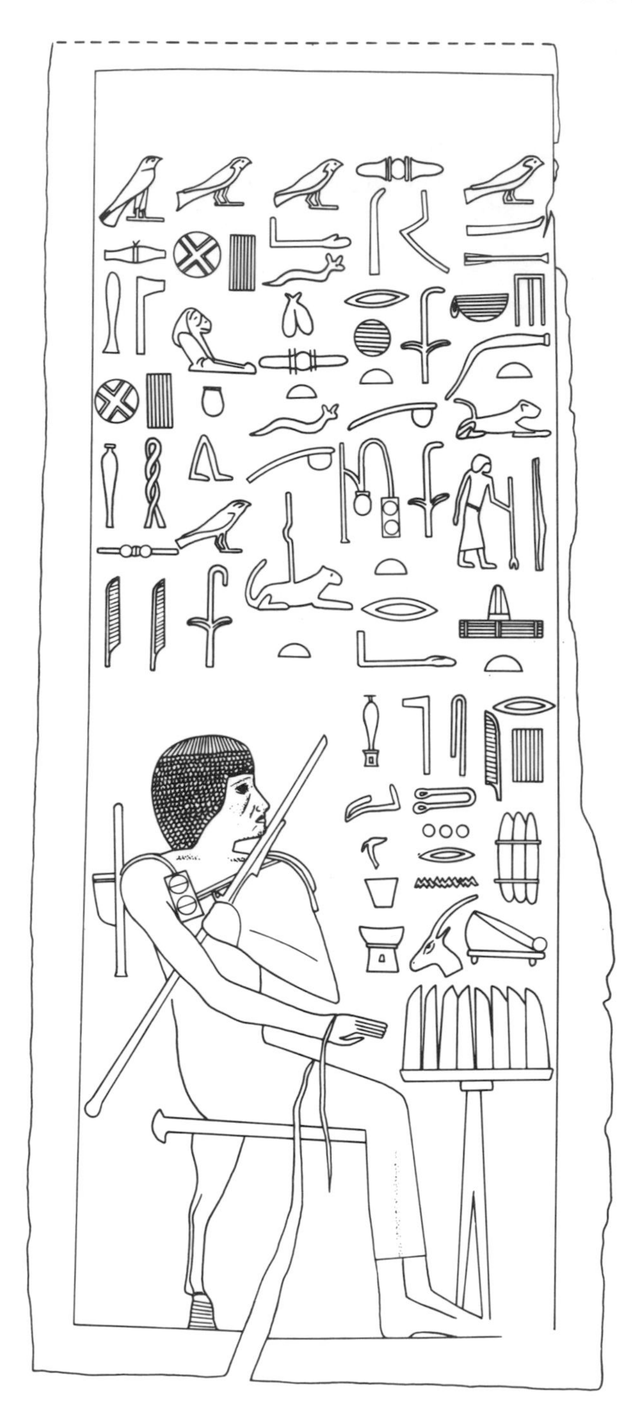

On his funeral stele, Nefer, a New Kingdom physician at the court of Amenophis I (1525–1504 B.C.), told why he deserved to enjoy his afterlife in the next world:

> *[I was] one on whom the north wind itself reaches, and one whose nose the wind is not prevented from [reaching], so that I may receive offerings, my heart being glad and joyful. I was the son of a mayor, a city nobleman and an overseer of the granaries of Amun in Karnak, energetic in going forth to the field of festival-food, [who spent his] old age in the favour of the king. [I] was one with whom [the king's]* ka *was pleased when the divine consort Ahmose-Nefertiry, justified with the great god lord of the West, flew to heaven [Nefer seems to have treated the king's mother]. I fare in my boat and moor at my plot of land. I plough with my oxen and bring in [my] corn on my asses. My goodly plot of land in the country which I cultivate was assigned to me in recognition of my valiant service; its produce becomes* htp-*bundles of divine offerings. I was one who was truly modest from the womb of my mother, one whom everyone would wish to be like. I did not rob the poor man on the road. I was friendly with the great. I did not defame my mother, my father did not find fault with me.* I am a truly excellent scribe, a dexterous physician who knows prescriptions which have many uses and who has investigated diseases of the body *[emphasis added]. I was a valiant warrior in my youth. I snared waterfowl and caught fish casting the net from my self-made boat.*[32]

Some of Nefer's claims may be only stock phrases, and the word translated as "investigated" should not be interpreted within the context of modern scientific medicine, but his statement exemplifies the life goals of a court physician—perhaps those of all courtiers.

Physicians in the royal service could be rewarded handsomely. The pharaoh Akhenaten (1353–1335 B.C.) gave a collar of gold to a *swnw* named Penthu. In fact, the walls of Penthu's tomb at Tell el-Amarna show him receiving the "collar of recognition" from a court official on three

FIGURE 5. One of several wooden panels from the Dynasty III tomb of Hesy-Rē. This one shows him sitting before an offering table piled with bread with a scribe's ink palette hanging over his right shoulder. The hieroglyphs list his many titles; the three hieroglyphs in the upper right corner identify him as a "chief tooth physician." Drawing by Yvonne Markowitz.

separate occasions.[33] The tomb of another New Kingdom physician, Neb-Amon, shows him being presented with valuable gifts by a Syrian prince.[34]

Most *swnw* did not, of course, work in the royal court. Nor did they anticipate being rewarded with gold, since virtually all financial transactions involved barter. The earliest Egyptian coins did not appear until Dynasty XXX (380–343 B.C.), long after the first contacts with Greek merchants had been made. However, at least by the New Kingdom, Egyptians usually valued commodities by the *deben*, a unit of weight (= 91 grams = 3.21 ounces) often expressed in terms of copper (but sometimes in silver). Occasionally they even paid debts with pieces of copper because the copper could be transported more easily than most bartered items; thus a *deben* of copper could function as a true coin. The other major unit of barter was the *khar*, a measure of capacity equivalent to 78.2 or 97.8 liters (= 20.7 or 25.8 gallons, or 2.6 and 3.2 bushels), most often used for grains.[35]

Physicians, like everyone else, were usually paid with food or other necessities of everyday life. In one Old Kingdom document, the unit of payment for their professional services was a loaf of bread or a pot of beer. Over the centuries other necessities of life became part of their wages, such as clothing, lodging, and other foods. Any excess over their immediate needs could then be bartered for other items the *swnw* wanted. In about 1274 B.C., during the reign of Ramesses II, two scribes and a physician at the royal necropolis at Thebes earned grain rations of one *khar* each (although for how much work was not specified), while a porter was given three;[36] the work of the *swnw* may not have been valued as highly as that of an unskilled laborer.

A papyrus dated about 1165 B.C. (Turin Papyrus no. 1880) provides the earliest known detailed list of payments to any physician:

Year 29 [of the reign of Ramesses III], fourth month of the inundation, last day;
that which is given to the physician by Userhat:
1 bronze ewer making 4 deben*;*
1 coiled basket making 5 deben*;*
2 pairs of sandals making 4 deben*;*
1 wooden rod [or staff] making ½ deben*;*
1 basket with lid making ¼ khar*;*
1 coiled basket making 5 deben*;*
Oil [possibly castor oil], 2 jars, making ½ khar*;*
Wooden object [possibly a small piece of furniture], making 2 deben*;*

> *Fine matting making ¼* khar;
> *Totalling 22* deben.[37]

At that time, a period of relative economic stability compared to the inflation of the preceding reigns, a *khar* of either barley or emmer wheat was usually valued at two copper *deben*,[38] but in this case the *khar* was worth 1½ *deben*. The exact reason for the payment was not stated in the document, although it was probably for professional services rendered. In any case, the total value of 22 *deben* is unexpectedly large; it would have been equivalent payment for a wooden bed or coffin, or for four goats. Because many *swnw* worked at palaces, quarries, necropolises, and in the army, it is also possible, in explaining the size of this payment, that Userhat was paying out some portion of the anonymous physician's regular wages for treating all who were injured or became sick at the work site, since his income probably did not depend simply on the number of patients he treated.[39]

Egyptian physicians had an enviable collective reputation throughout the ancient world. Niqmad, king of Ugarit, a city on the northeast Mediterranean, wrote to the pharaoh Akhenaten around 1350 B.C. to ask for two Nubian court pages and "a palace physician [because] we have no physicians here."[40] A century later, king Hattusili of the Hittites wrote to ask his son-in-law Ramesses II to send help for an unusual—and, as the pharaoh knew, insoluble—medical problem. The Egyptian king's reply is almost insulting:

> *[You] would like me to send a man to prepare for [your sister]*
> *a drug to let her be with child . . .*
> *Is she fifty years old? Nonsense!*
> *She is sixty.*
> *And see, a woman fifty years old,*
> *No! one who is sixty,*
> *One cannot prepare for her a drug*
> *To let her be with child.*
> *Indeed, the Sun god and the Weather god [the major Hittite deities] may—to please her—*
> *Issue an order and the dispositions thereof*
> *Will be lastingly dispensed to her*
> *And I, the King, your Brother,*
> *Will send you an able exorciser priest and an able physician.*
> *And they will prepare to her intent drugs*
> *So that she [will] be with child.*[41]

On other occasions, however, Ramesses was less sarcastic. He sent drugs—but not a physician—for the Hittite king's eye problems, and promised to send a *swnw*, and perhaps an exorcist priest, to drive out a disease-producing demon. But then the pharaoh had to ask his father-in-law to obtain the release of two *swnw* who had been sent to, and then forcibly detained at, the court of a powerful Hittite nobleman.[42]

Seven centuries later, Herodotus told how Persian monarchs liked to have Egyptian physicians at their courts. For instance, before the Persians conquered Egypt, the pharaoh Amasis (570–526 B.C.) honored Cambyses' request to send him an eye specialist. Unfortunately, the ancient ophthalmologist was so angered at being torn away from his family that he contrived the situation that led to Egypt's subjection by Persia. (However, this story is likely to have been, at best, an exaggeration.) Darius, Cambyses' successor, liked to have Egyptian physicians at his court, although he nearly executed them all by impalement when a Greek physician cured him of an ailment that they had failed to cure.[43]

It seems fair to conclude that physicians were held in high esteem in ancient Egypt, although only those at the royal court were lavishly rewarded. As will be seen later, much of their reputation probably originated in their association with the learned scribal tradition, or in their bureaucratic services for, and friendships with, their kings, rather than in their skills as healers. Still, some foreign monarchs tried to recruit Egyptian healers to their own courts. But in the end, it was the Egyptian people—royalty or commoners—whom the *swnw* were most often called upon to treat.

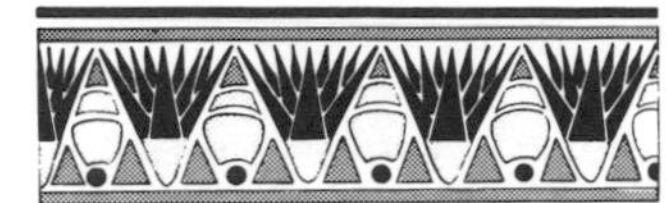

2

THE EGYPTIANS AND THEIR DISEASES: THE ARCHAEOLOGICAL EVIDENCE

About 27 centuries after Imhotep invented the pyramid, the Roman scholar Pliny the Elder reported that the Egyptians thought they had invented the arts and skills of medicine.[1] They probably were the first to write about the subject, but it does not seem reasonable to suppose that theirs was the first culture to concern itself with pain, wounds, illness, and the prevention of death.

If all the surviving written sources for ancient Egyptian medicine were to be translated into English, they could be printed in one modest-sized volume, although several more volumes would be required for critical annotations. Hundreds of pages of exegesis are already in print in both the Egyptological and medical historical literature. This chapter will be concerned chiefly with the archaeological and ecological evidence pertaining to health, disease, death, and other aspects of everyday life on the Nile, in order to provide a background against which the medical papyri and other ancient views of illness can be interpreted. The next three chapters will introduce the contents of those papyri and supplement them with other ancient views of health and disease.

The geography and probably the disease patterns familiar to the *swnw* were, by modern standards, extraordinarily constant over time and along the entire length of the Nile from Aswan to the sea. The extent of the water table on either side of its pathway through the desert restricted the habitable and arable portion of Upper Egypt to a 550-mile long strip that narrowed from about 30 miles wide near Memphis to less than a mile wide at the southern boundary. Lower Egypt, the delta, comprised the other half of the kingdom's agricultural land. Since rainfall was minimal throughout the country, Egypt's agricultural success, based on multitudinous local irrigation ditch systems, was one of her major accomplishments.[2]

Food production was facilitated, of course, by the usually dependable regularity of the Nile's annual inundations, which deposited fertile silt along the river's entire course. The Egyptians always feared low floods, but their actual frequency has been difficult to ascertain. Drought-induced famine does seem to have contributed to political instability throughout the century called the First Intermediate Period (2134–2040 B.C.), between the Old and Middle Kingdoms. Conversely, no famines or low floods are recorded for Dynasty XVIII, a high point in the history of pharaonic power.[3]

Archaeologists and anthropologists can usually rely on any of several indices to assess the overall health of ancient populations. The simplest is longevity, while estimates of growth rate and nutritional status must depend on more indirect data, such as stature and other skeletal measurements (including some that can be made only by radiography), the concentration of certain trace elements in bone, dental studies, the detection of specific pathological lesions in preserved bodies, and the proportion of births to childhood deaths.

Evidence from around the eastern Mediterranean basin (although few of the data come from Egypt) has shown that as prehistoric populations in that general area evolved from nomadic hunter-gatherers into more sedentary agricultural village-dwellers their nutritional status and growth rates declined for a variety of reasons. One was the decreased amount of animal protein in their diet as hunting was abandoned as a way of life. However, once irrigation systems had been installed, beginning in Predynastic times, grains and then many other new foods could be incorporated into the standard Egyptian diet. As a result, stature, longevity, and overall health began to revert toward their earlier maxima. The Egyptians achieved their peak productivity, and probably peak health status, during the New Kingdom, followed by a further peak under Roman rule.[4]

Probably because cereals and vegetables came to make up as much as 90 percent of the usual diet, and to replace the dietary contributions of red meat, stature (an index of protein intake) fell as one result of the

Agricultural Revolution. It has been postulated that only since the beginning of the Industrial Revolution have we begun to approach the average height of our hunter-gatherer ancestors. The wild game available in prehistoric Africa in their day contained far less fat, and more of the polyunsaturated fatty acids thought to protect against atherosclerosis (fatty deposits in arteries), than in modern domestic livestock. The average diet of late Paleolithic North Africans included about 35 percent meat and 65 percent vegetable foods. By the early Old Kingdom, most Egyptians probably ate something like 80 percent of their diet as carbohydrates, largely grain, 10 percent as fat, and only 10 percent as animal protein (although some protein is, of course, found in cereal grains). Additional sources of carbohydrate calories included wine for the rich and beer for peasants. Beer, made from barley sprouts and fermented for only one day with partially baked bread, contained more alcohol than the 6 percent typical of modern American beers, although intemperance was regarded as immoral by almost everyone, rich and poor. Dietary supplies of iron, vitamins, and essential minerals were probably adequate, on the whole.[5]

Food, sustenance

Red meats were consumed only infrequently in Dynastic Egypt, largely because of their scarcity, but also because some animals associated with specific gods were taboo. For instance, the lepidotus fish (*Barbus binni*) was proscribed because it was sacred to Osiris, the god of the dead, whose form was taken by all Egyptians in the afterlife. (However, other taboo species, such as the highly revered oxyrhynchus fish [*Mormyrus kannume*], were sometimes eaten anyway.) Beef was limited chiefly to the elite class, as were several species of wild game such as rabbits and the various African antelopes. The average Egyptian was more likely to eat goat, an occasional ibex, and, less frequently, sheep and pork. The richer food served at royal and provincial courts may account for the cases of atherosclerosis seen in mummies of the well-to-do. Fish, caught by hand, or with hooks, traps, nets, and spears, was an important source of animal protein, especially for the poor. The most frequently portrayed Nile fish species included the bolti (*Tilapia nilotica*), *Synodontis schall*, and the mullet (*Mugil cephalus*). If not cooked and eaten immediately, they could be sun-dried for future use. Fowl were among the other sources of animal protein; some were domesticated, especially geese, ducks, doves, and pigeons (but not chickens), while nets and snares were used to catch exotic wild birds. Eggs were probably not part of the Egyptian diet, although they were included in several drug mixtures.[6]

Domesticated cereals were introduced into Egypt during the Neolithic era. The Agricultural Revolution began with barley (*Hordeum vulgare* or *H. hexastichum*) and emmer wheat (*Triticum dicoccum*). Both flourished so well along the Nile that, many centuries later, the Romans realized that annexation of the whole country could help feed the city of Rome, among other potential benefits. Flour was ground by hand with stone implements that left tiny abrasive particles in the flour. Not only pictures but also actual specimens of breads have survived from all periods of Egyptian history. They were prepared in many shapes and sizes, from a wide variety of recipes; some were sweetened with dates or other fruits, or with honey, the only sweetening agents used in pharaonic Egypt.[7]

Among the common edible vegetables were several legumes that probably contributed to the Egyptians' protein intake, especially broad beans (*Vicia faba*), chick peas (*Cicer arietum*), lentils (*Ervum lens*), common peas (*Pisum sativum*), and the Egyptian bean or pink lotus (*Nelumbium speciosum* or *Nymphaea nelumbo*); samples of most have been found preserved in tombs. Other green vegetables known to have been prominent in the diet were the onion, garlic, and leek (*Allium cepa, A. sativum*, and *A. porrum*, respectively), cabbage (*Brassica oleracea*), celery (*Apium graveolens*), lettuce (*Lactuca sativa*), and cucumber (*Cucumis sativus*). Tubers of the sedge (*Cyperus esculenta*) and the soft parts of papyrus stems (*Cyperus papyrus*) were also eaten. Many fruits and nuts were introduced in succession throughout pharaonic history, presumably as contacts were made with other countries. Among the most important indigenous fruits was the date palm (*Phoenix dactylifera*), a major source of carbohydrate because it generally produces 40 to 80 kilograms (88–176 pounds) of fruit each year, containing 50 percent sugar by weight. Other native fruits included the sycomore fig or Egyptian mulberry (*Ficus sycomorus*), the dom palm (*Hyphaena thebaica*), and the jujube (*Zizyphus spina-Christi*). Old Kingdom additions to the Egyptian menu included the fig (*Ficus caricus*), grapes and raisins (*Vitis vinifera*), the kernels of the hegelig thorn tree (*Balanites aegyptica*), and the persea (*Mimusops schimperi*). Pomegranates (*Punica granatum*) and probably the carob (*Ceratonia siliqua*) first appeared during the Middle Kingdom, and, in the New Kingdom, the Egyptian plum (*Cordia myxa*), olive (*Olea europea*), watermelon (*Citrullus vulgaris*), and apple (*Malus sylvestris*). The cultivation of cherries, citrons, peaches, and pears was introduced by the Greeks and Romans.[8]

Infants lived largely on their mothers' milk until they were weaned at the age of three, although other foods were, presumably, added to their diet before then. The extent to which cow's, goat's, or other milks, butter, and cheese were used is not clear, although it does seem to have grown over the centuries. Animal fats (e.g., beef, ibex, and goose) and vegetable oils (especially oil from the ben tree, *Moringa aptera*, and olive oil) entered Egyptian kitchens during the New Kingdom, as did a wide range of spices and herbs.[9]

The typical Early Dynastic diet consisted of leavened breads, soups and porridges made with legumes, perhaps other vegetables, dates, and beer. Fish, milk, several fruits, and cheese were added to this basic repertoire during the Old Kingdom; most domesticated animals were reserved for utilitarian purposes such as transportation and plowing, and perhaps for milking. The rather sumptuous menu placed in the tomb of a minor noblewoman of Dynasty II (2770–2649 B.C.) at Sakkara included a barley porridge, loaves and cakes made of emmer wheat, a cooked quail, pigeon stew, kidneys, ribs of beef, fish, stewed fruit, fresh berries, cheese, wine, and possibly beer. The New Kingdom saw an expansion of the overall food supply and the introduction of new ways of cooking and preserving many foods, especially with fats, oils, and added flour, and new fruits and vegetables appeared. One modern estimate of the standard daily ration for a quarry worker is 1.8 kilograms (4 pounds) of bread, although he was surely given other foods as well, while soldiers received bread, vegetables, onions, beef, cakes, and beer, but the amount and frequency of each were not reported. The rations for people in all workplaces ranged from as low as 1200 calories per day, to the usual 3000, on up to a probable maximum of 5000.[10]

All in all, the diet of the average Egyptian, rich or poor, was probably balanced among the basic food groups, and it may have filled his caloric needs, but not much more. There is little evidence of either obesity or unnecessary luxuries in ancient Egypt, although high officials from as early as the Old Kingdom liked to have themselves portrayed with enough abdominal fat to indicate how prosperous they were. By contrast, the ordinary farm or construction worker probably burned off most of the calories he ingested in his usual three meals a day (courtiers had five). Diet was probably as varied as economic and agricultural circumstances would allow, and it almost certainly filled basic requirements for the complete range of vitamins and minerals, although salt intake was far less than ours. On a typical New Kingdom stele, a royal overseer named Amen-em-Hab and his wife are shown sitting before a table piled high with food. A prayer, which summarizes the wealthier Egyptian's basic dietary needs, asks that the deceased be granted a similarly bountiful table, with "bread and beer, beef and fowl, libations, wine, milk and everything good and pure."[11]

Taxes in kind left most Egyptians—who were, by and large, farmers—with little excess food to store in their own granaries as protection against famine. Because most surplus food was stored by the central government, civil war or mere political instability could result in widespread hunger, especially when irrigation systems also failed. Most kings probably recognized the relationships among food supply, workers' productivity, and civil unrest; Ramesses II was quoted as saying that laborers perform best "when the belly is satisfied." The potential impact of famine is dramatized in the familiar tale (*Genesis 41–45*) of Joseph's rise to power (perhaps in a New Kingdom court). Probably because recorded famines are so few, we lack detailed demographic evidence of their actual effects on Egyptians.[12]

However, they knew what to expect. An inscription on a granite rock on Sehel Island near Aswan, written during the Ptolemaic period (although it purports to be a Dynasty III decree by Zoser), portrays a famine caused by the Nile's failure to flood adequately:

I [Zoser] was in mourning on my throne,
Those of the palace were in grief,
My heart was in great affliction,
Because Hapy [the Nile] had failed to come in time
In a period of seven years.
Grain was scant,
Kernels were dried up,
Scarce was every kind of food.
Every man robbed his twin,
Those who entered [a house] did not go [out of it because they were too weak with hunger].
Children cried,
Youngsters fell,
The hearts of the old were grieving;
Legs drawn up, they hugged the ground,
Their arms clasped about them.
Courtiers were needy,
Temples were shut,

Shrines covered with dust,
Everyone was in distress.[13]

Even if this inscription does not portray an actual Old Kingdom famine, a relief carved at Sakkara, on the funerary causeway of Unas (2356–2323 B.C.), the last king of Dynasty V, probably does. It shows grotesquely emaciated men and women whose prominent ribs taper down to their narrow waists and bony hips. Although these victims are not portrayed as typical ethnic Egyptians, they are clearly meant to represent the effects of serious famine.[14]

During the difficult times of the First Intermediate Period, one nomarch, or provincial governor, managed the resources of his district so well—or so he said in his tomb inscriptions—that "death from hunger never happened in this nome," although "the whole of Upper Egypt died from famine [to the extent that] all men ate their children." A century later, around 2000 B.C., a farmer who lived near Thebes scolded his family for complaining about the short rations they were receiving because of a recent poor harvest. He pointed out that in some parts of Egypt, there were no rations at all, and that "They are beginning to eat men here." Both references to cannibalism are probably more rhetorical than real, but they underline the Egyptians' worst fears of famine. At the same time, the evidence from the governor and the farmer suggests that good management of whatever food resources were available could help Egyptians pull through such disasters.[15]

Thus, although Egypt's soil could be richly productive, her people's life was precariously based on the necessity for irrigation farming. Moreover, the valley was not uniformly settled, and towns tended to appear and disappear over the centuries as long-term flooding patterns changed. It has been estimated that Egyptian farmers produced 1650 pounds of wheat or 1560 pounds of barley per acre, which could supply just over one pound of grain per person per day during the New Kingdom.[16] That amount is consistent with the rations cited earlier, but it still provided only marginally sufficient nutrition.

The total population of Egypt fell by about a third in the probably drought-stricken last years of both the Old and New Kingdoms, and by about a sixth after Alexander's conquest. Figure 6 provides an overview of the slowly changing human ecosystems of the Nile valley and delta. The calculated and somewhat hypothetical data used to construct the graph show that through the end of the Old Kingdom population density increased steadily, as more and more land was brought under irrigation and cultivation. Also during that time, the population density in the valley

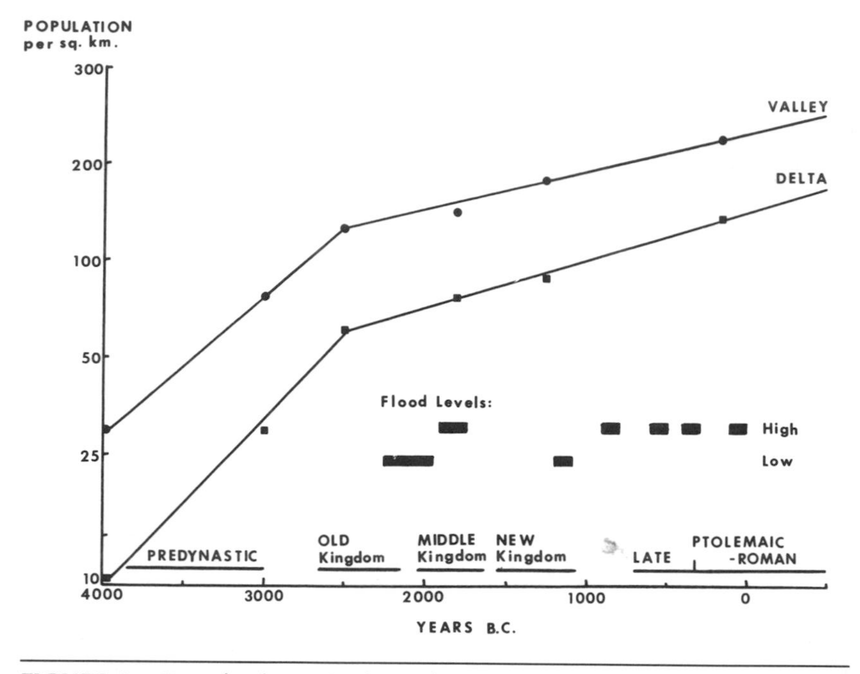

FIGURE 6. Growth of estimated population density in the Nile Valley and the Nile Delta. Data for the country as a whole, including people who lived in the desert and the Faiyum (a very large oasis area), fall on a line intermediate between those shown here; the total population of Egypt in 1882, the date of the first modern census before the first Aswan dam (1902) made it possible to feed more people than ever before, lies on the straight line that can be extrapolated from the data for the country as a whole before the year 1 A.D. This suggests that the relationship between agricultural methods and population remained relatively constant from 2500 B.C. until 1900 A.D. Later improvements in the country's ability to feed itself have by now vastly increased the population density out of proportion to its historical trends up until 1902. The periods of low and high Nile floods are estimates at best. SOURCE: Karl W. Butzer, *Early Hydraulic Civilization in Egypt: a Study in Cultural Ecology* (Chicago, 1976): 25-33, 51, 82-89.

doubled approximately every 715 years, and in the delta every 587 years. Low floods brought more frequent famines for 300 years beginning near the end of the Old Kingdom, when the famine victims were portrayed at the funerary complex of Unas. These repetitive, although not necessarily constant, droughts must have destabilized the kingdom throughout the First Intermediate Period, just as low floods did for a century at the end of the New Kingdom, although no serious famines are recorded for that time. But the Middle and New Kingdoms were also ravaged for many years running by exceptionally high floods. They destroyed not only food stores, livestock, and population, but also buildings and the vital irrigation systems, requiring extensive labor (and calories) to rebuild them. In addition, prolonged dampness favored the proliferation of plant parasites, which fed on the crops that managed to survive. After 2500 B.C., the population density doubled more slowly than before, about every 2524 years in the valley and every 2004 years in the delta. It is hazardous to ascribe the much slower population growth rates after the Old Kingdom solely to irregular Nile floods, but they must have contributed to the overall decrease.[17]

It might have been assumed, albeit intuitively, that both low and high floods must have produced epidemics, or at least widespread disease burdens, in ancient Egypt, although there is virtually no contemporary evidence for major devastating plagues. A few texts, such as the one anachronistically attributed to Zoser, focus on famine instead. Indeed, it has been postulated that many infectious agents, especially those that do not require nonhuman hosts as vectors, simply cannot cause significant mortality in human populations that are insufficiently dense to permit the micro-organisms to continue spreading to new hosts in which they can multiply further. In the absence of their necessary human hosts, many bacteria and viruses must have succumbed to the desiccating force of the Egyptian environment. Until relatively recent times, the chief pathologic checks on human population growth have been the acute infectious diseases of childhood, but many of them may not have caused demographically significant mortality in early man.[18] Instead, it was probably nonbacterial and nonviral parasites with animal reservoirs, such as schistosomiasis and hookworm, that caused the highest morbidity and mortality on the banks of the Nile, along with tuberculosis, which is an insidiously fatal bacterial disease, not an acute or quickly life-threatening one.

If serious epidemics of dramatically acute illnesses were not prominent in the lives of ancient Egyptians—however improbable that seems—then we can infer that their food supply, population density, mortality rate, and average life expectancy were even more closely correlated than they have been in Europe and America since the seventeenth century.[19] It has also been hypothesized that crowding, by reducing available food resources, results not only in an increased death rate but also in a general decline in fertility as nutritional needs go unmet.[20]

The late Palaeolithic peoples of Nubia were hunter-gatherers who obtained their food with more difficulty than the agriculturalists of Dynastic Egypt experienced. Consequently, the Nubians' life expectancy at birth, as determined from skeletal remains in cemeteries, was shorter than that of later Egyptians, but the rate of increase of life expectancy at birth over the ensuing centuries seems to have been similar among both peoples (see Figure 7). Nubian men tended to outlive women, at least up to

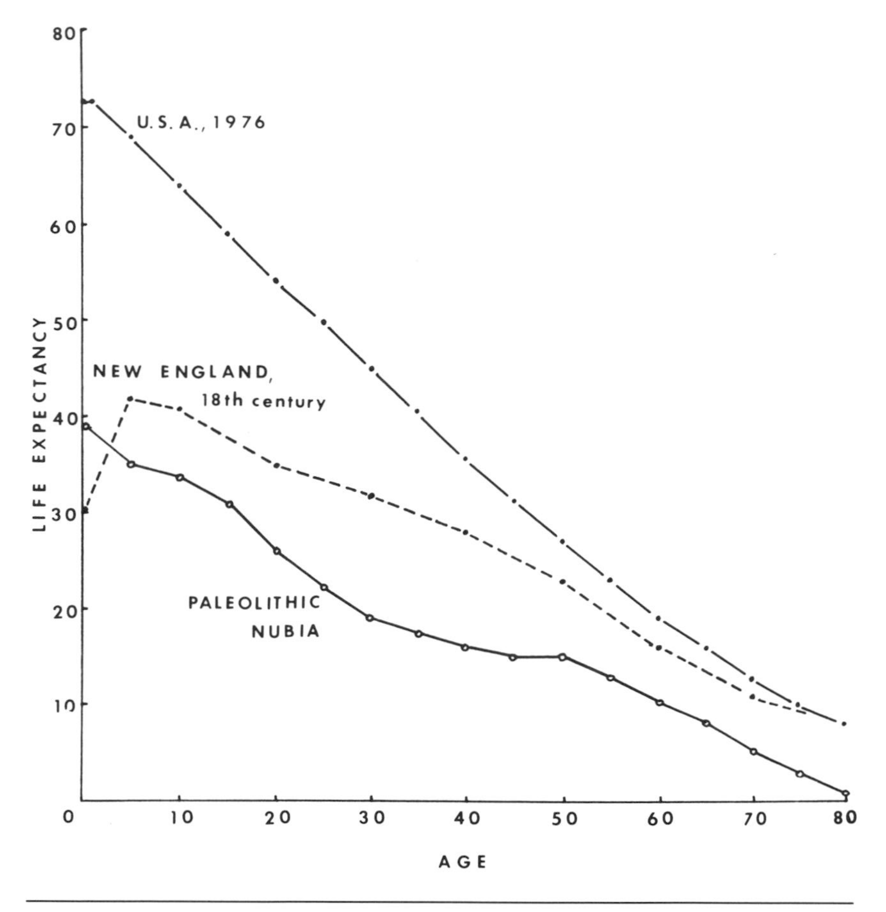

FIGURE 7. Average life expectancy in Paleolithic Nubia, compared with data for modern America and eighteenth-century New England. SOURCES: *Facts of Life and Death* (U.S. Department of Health, Education, and Welfare Publication No. [PHS] 79-1222, 1978), 6; J. Worth Estes, *Hall Jackson and the Purple Foxglove: Medical Practice and Research in Revolutionary America, 1760-1820* (Hanover, N.H., 1979), 126-129; J. Nemeskéri, "Some Comparisons of Egyptian and Early Eurasian Demographic Data," *Journal of Human Evolution 1* (1972): 171-186.

the age of 40 (see Figure 8).[21] Such data have led to the conclusion that childbearing was dangerous to women's health;[22] this hypothesis can be buttressed indirectly by a few data from Predynastic and Dynastic Egypt, but it cannot be confirmed from independent sources.

Average life expectancy at birth has been difficult to estimate even from the remains uncovered in Egyptian cemeteries. Because most of these cemeteries lack substantial numbers of infant and adolescent skel-

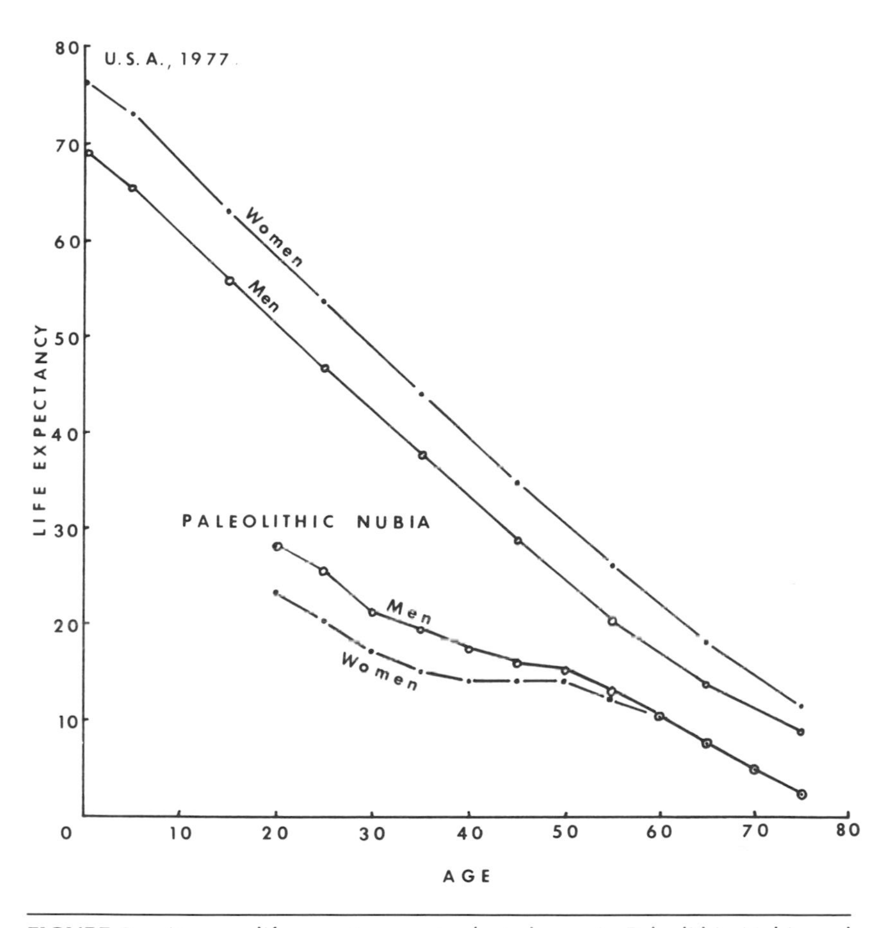

FIGURE 8. Average life expectancy at selected ages in Paleolithic Nubia and modern America by sex. SOURCES: Metropolitan Life Insurance Company, *Statistical Bulletin 61*, no. 2 (April-June 1980), 2; Nemeskéri, "Demographic Data," see Figure 7.

etons, they are not adequate random samples, or cross-sections, of the population. The average age at death among 709 adult Egyptian skulls at Turin, Italy, has been estimated at about 30 years for Predynastic adults and 36 years from the Old Kingdom onward. Although the data provide no clues to life expectancy at birth, since no children's skulls were included in the sample, they do suggest that fewer than 10 percent of Predynastic Egyptians lived more than 40 years, or more than 50 years in Dynastic times. (By contrast, about 94 percent of modern Americans survive their fortieth birthdays.) Other data support the general conclusion that life expectancy increased from about 25–30 years during Palaeolithic and Neolithic times to about 35–40 by the New Kingdom, and that much of the earlier high mortality was probably ascribable to a higher proportion of Palaeolithic infant deaths, even if we lack the pathological specimens necessary to confirm that hypothesis.[23] It can probably be taken as axiomatic that the odds of surviving those diseases that were most prominent in ancient Egypt were greatest when the body's nutritional requirements for fighting off such illnesses were most fully satisfied. The absence of positive confirmation from the mummified remains of children and adults precludes finding proof of a clearcut cause-effect relationship. Nevertheless, the apparent gradual increase in agricultural productivity may well be related to increased life expectancy during the Dynastic period.

X-rays have provided reliable estimates of the ages of the royal mummies in the Egyptian Museum at Cairo. The results can be compared with estimates of their life spans derived from written evidence (plus that for three kings and three queens who were not X-rayed). In general the ages of death estimated by both methods are similar. The perhaps more reliable radiographic measurements of skeletal age show that 40 percent of the New Kingdom pharaohs died in their early thirties and 8 percent after the age of 45. Because radiological signs of the aging process stabilize by about the age of 50, it is necessary to rely on written records for Ramesses II (1290–1224 B.C.) and his son Merneptah (1224–1214 B.C.), who are known to have been about 92 and 70, respectively, when they died. Difficulties in interpreting the historical texts undoubtedly account for the relatively minor discrepancies between them and the more objective data revealed by X-rays in the other cases.[24]

When taken in aggregate, the few data we do have can probably permit the conclusion that one-half of Dynastic Egyptians died by the age of about 34, and 90 percent by the age of 50, although some did reach age 90 or more. Those who lived longest were usually members of the privileged classes. However, even if extreme longevity was achieved by very few Egyptians, they still thought of it as a desirable reward for good living—110 years seems to have been a favorite goal.[25] For purposes of comparison, in 1917–1927 the Egyptians' mean life expectancy at birth was 31 years for men and 36 years for women; by 1969 those values had increased to 51.6 and 53.8 years, respectively.[26] (Life expectancy was 71.2 and 78.2 years for American men and women, respectively, in 1985.)

The average age at marriage was 15 to 20 for men and 12 to 13 for their wives, although it is not clear that women so young were able to bear children. Only for Ptolemaic queens has the average fertility rate been estimated, about 3.6 live births per woman. Low fertility rates may even have helped maintain the balance between the size of the population (especially at the provincial level) and its food resources, permitting the population to increase most when the food supply was most abundant. Egyptians considered themselves to be technically children until the age of five, and a "young person" was defined as one between age five and 16, after which his age began to be counted. The usual three-year lactation period may have contributed to minimizing the fertility rate, although women can become pregnant after they have been nursing for some time. Reduced nutrition, as in time of famine, would also tend to inhibit reproduction.[27]

Egyptians of all classes (except priests) could have more than one wife at a time, at least in the form of legal concubines, although it would seem that only the elite could afford such luxuries. Prostitution was not approved, and adultery was punished, but Egyptians were not especially prudish when it came to clothing or to representing the body in art. However, a man who masturbated or committed a homosexual act risked not winning entrance to the netherworld, perhaps because such behavior indicated weakness of character, and several provinces found it necessary to outlaw sodomy. Still, a charm for attracting another man has survived from Roman Egypt, as well as one a woman could use to seduce another woman.[28]

The inhabitants of Dynastic Egypt were about six inches shorter than modern Americans; men averaged 61.8 inches (157 centimeters) in height, and women 58.3 inches (148 centimeters). Because Dynastic men were 3.2 inches shorter than their Predynastic forefathers, and women 3.5 inches shorter than their Predynastic counterparts, it may be inferred that their stature diminished as the Egyptians abandoned hunting for the less rigorous life of the farmer. On the other hand, many texts and tomb pictures show that the labor-intensive agricultural life demanded great expenditure of energy—and, therefore, of calories—so the relative paucity of red meat proteins may have been a relatively greater contributor to loss of stature among Dynastic Egyptians. X-rays of mummies often reveal skeletal evidence of episodes of childhood illnesses in the form of "arrested growth lines" (also called Harris lines), which indicate that bone growth has temporarily slowed or halted while the youngster's body fended off infections. The high prevalence of such evidence in skeletal remains from many Egyptian tombs and cemeteries indirectly suggests that the comparative safety and stability that accompanied the shift from nomadism to farming may have permitted more children to survive childhood, but, at the same time, children's diseases may have reduced their final achievable height. However, the rate (velocity) at which children grew to their adult stature was about the same in prehistoric Nubia as in modern America.[29]

Most of the available data pertaining to the Egyptians' stature have been published in forms that preclude appropriate statistical assessments of its variations. However, the heights of the Egyptians do seem to have been somewhat more homogeneous than those of modern Americans, probably because of Americans' far greater genetic diversity. If the ancient Egyptians' gene pool was actually more homogeneous than ours, it may have been because they were extremely unlikely to marry people from other countries. Consanguinity may have been another contributory factor, inasmuch as many texts tell of marriages between "brother" and "sister." However, although such matings sometimes did occur within royal families, they were far less frequent among commoners; the words "brother" and "sister" were often used simply as synonyms for husbands and wives, or as terms of endearment.[30] The hypothesis that the population of the ancient Nile valley shared many genes in common is also supported by evidence that their blood group gene frequencies remained relatively stable over some 5000 years,[31] as is generally true for inbred populations. The ancient Egyptians appear to have been distinguished by a high frequency of genes for blood group B; it is less frequent today.[32]

Mummy

Mummification was essentially a desiccation process. It evolved over several centuries after the earliest Egyptians first observed that the naked body was more or less preserved after its customary burial in relatively shallow pits in the hot dry sand. In its full development, which persisted until about 300–400 A.D., mummification was accomplished with natron, a naturally occurring mixture of sodium salts, chiefly the carbonate and bicarbonate. Modern experiments with the carcasses of laboratory animals have helped ascertain the optimum proportions of dry natron that were probably packed into body cavities. Unguents and resins were then applied to the skin surface and just below it to provide additional strengthening and preservative properties. For religious and philosophical reasons, the heart was usually left *in situ*.[33]

So were the kidneys and organs adjacent to them, but they were probably left behind chiefly because embalmers, reaching blindly into the abdomen, could not easily feel them, since the kidneys lie in the retroperitoneal space, between the fibrous rear wall of the abdominal cavity and the muscles of the back. The kidneys are not even mentioned in the surviving medical papyri. The other large organs were removed and preserved separately in four especially designated "canopic" jars, each capped by a carved head associated with one of the four sons of Horus: liver (human head, Amset); lungs (baboon head, Hapi); stomach (jackal head, Duamutef); and intestines (falcon head, Kebehsenuef). From the time of Ramesses V (1156–1151 B.C.) until the Late Period (712–332 B.C.), those organs were wrapped separately and then placed between the legs or in the abdomen; the use of canopic jars was resumed in Dynasty XXX (380–343 B.C.). By the advent of the Middle Kingdom, embalmers had begun to remove the brain altogether, usually through the nose, because as far as the Egyptians knew, it had neither physiological nor philosophical functions.

In the early nineteenth century of our era, the first mummies to appear in western European cities became objects of scientific investigation. In 1825 Dr. A. B. Granville dissected a female mummy (see Figure 9) before the Royal Society. He thought she had died before the pyramids were built, but she seems to date from sometime between the New Kingdom and Alexander's conquest in 332 B.C. Granville concluded that the woman, who was just over five feet tall, had had several pregnancies, and that she had died at about the age of 50–55 from ovarian dropsy (which, in 1825, usually meant a large cystic tumor of the ovary).[34]

Within ten years Dr. Thomas Joseph Pettigrew, also of London, had examined mummies in museums all over Europe, and one in his own collection. He found little in the way of recognizable pathology in any of them, although he dissected only two or three. One did show signs of healing around a fracture in the back of his skull, so he must have lived for some days after the presumably fatal wound was inflicted. But Pettigrew was more interested in using the techniques of physical an-

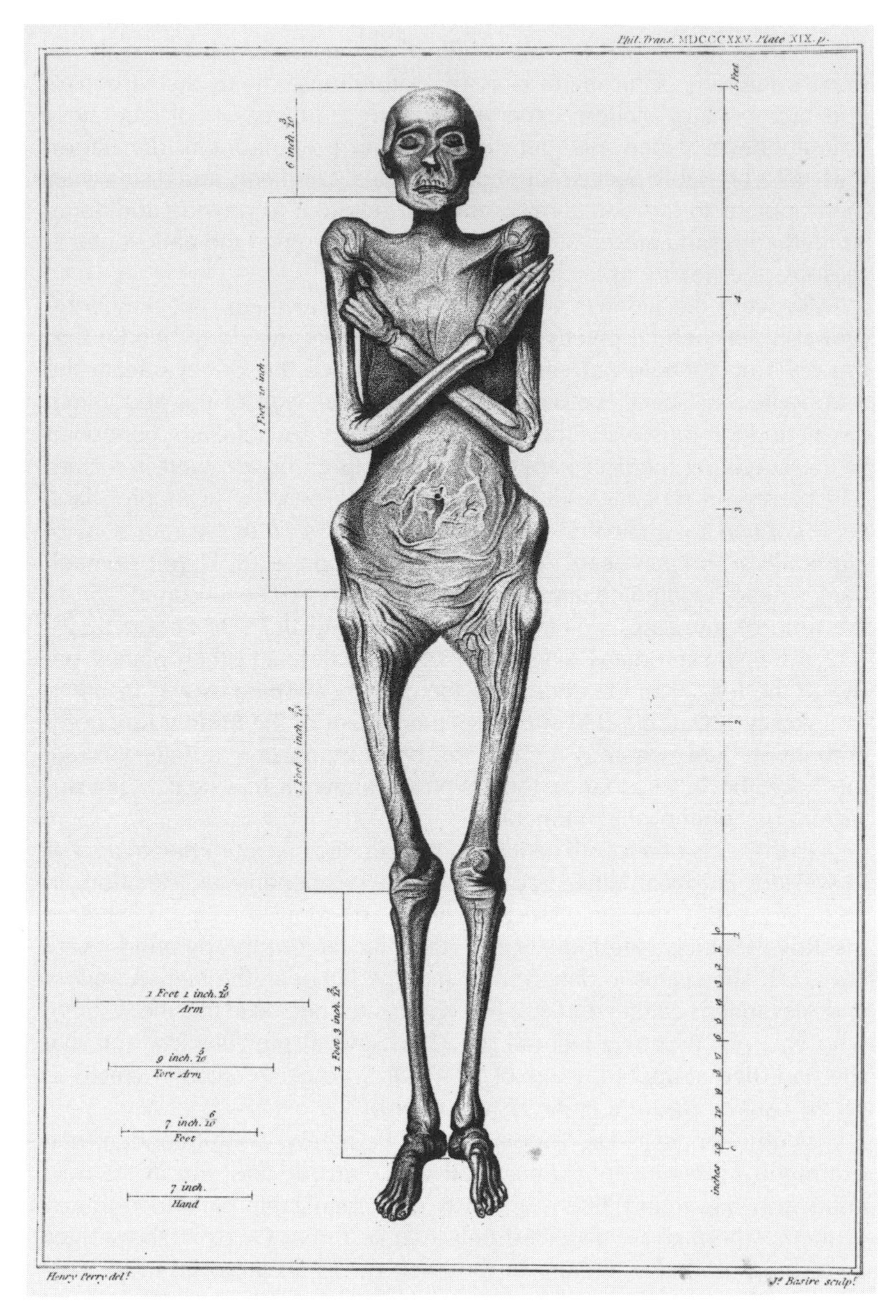
Phil. Trans. MDCCCXXV. Plate XIX. p.
6 inch. 3/10
1 Feet 10 inch.
1 Feet 5 inch. 2/10
1 Feet 3 inch. 2/10
1 Feet 1 inch. 5/10
Arm
9 inch. 5/10
Fore Arm
7 inch. 6/10
Foot
7 inch.
Hand
5 Feet
inches
Henry Perry del.
Js Basire sculp.

thropology to classify ancient Egyptians into racial types based on facial bone structure and height, so he did not pursue his pathological studies in any great detail.[35]

Several twentieth-century students of mummies have conducted far more careful investigations, although some published reports make any systematic analysis of the findings extremely difficult. In general, they have not revealed as much information as might have been anticipated, largely because the mummification process itself destroyed most of the microscopic detail that is necessary for making tissue diagnoses, especially of infectious diseases. However, noninvasive, or nondestructive methods, such as radiography, have provided additional clues to the Egyptians' health and diseases.

Sick people (literally, "diseased ones")

For instance, most of 78 British Museum mummies examined by X-ray were less than 40 years old when they died; 30 percent were children. The adults ranged around the usual five feet in height, and most showed radiographic evidence, in the form of arrested growth lines, of severe but unspecified illness during childhood. Many bones were fractured or dislocated post-mortem when embalmers tried to fit the finished mummies into coffins that were too small for them, as has been found in other mummies as well. The only diagnosable cause of death discovered among the British Museum "patients" was a severe skull fracture. Signs of osteoarthritis (also known as degenerative arthritis) were seen in 15 spines, as well as single cases each of spina bifida (failure of the lower end of the spine to close around the spinal cord during fetal development) and

---

FIGURE 9. Engraving of a female mummy dissected before the Royal Society in London in 1825. The woman, who was just over five feet tall, had had several pregnancies and died of a right ovarian tumor at the age of 50 to 55, during the last few centuries B.C. The abdominal contents had been rather clumsily removed through the anus, and the brain through the nostrils, but the muscles and thoracic organs were relatively well preserved, in the dissector's opinion. From A. B. Granville, *An Essay on Egyptian Mummies* (London, 1825). (Courtesy, Boston Medical Library)

osteogenesis imperfecta (an inherited disorder of bone structure that usually results in early death associated with multiple fractures). One man was found to have been circumcised; small, probably asymptomatic, gallstones were seen in another mummy; and arterial calcification, a sign of advanced arteriosclerosis, was seen in five others.[36]

X-ray studies of 29 royal mummies in the Cairo Museum revealed similar findings, although growth arrest lines were present in only three, as might be expected among the royal family. None showed any evidence of healed fractures, but one pharaoh, Seqenenre Tao (died about 1560 B.C.), probably perished on the battlefield from his severe skull wounds. Evidence of osteoarthritis was observed in all the royal mummies, and of ankylosing spondylitis (a form of rheumatoid arthritis in the spine seen primarily in men) in one, Amenhotep II (1427–1401 B.C.). The deformed left foot of Siptah (1204–1198 B.C.) very strongly suggests that he had had poliomyelitis earlier in his life, although it could have been a congenital clubfoot deformity called talipes equinovarus. Three royal women had marked scoliosis (lateral curvature of the spine). Several pharaohs showed extensive calcified atherosclerosis; two were among the longest-lived of all those examined.[37]

A few nonroyal ancient "patients" show clear evidence of healed fractures of the long bones in the leg and wrist. One young child died of fractures of the skull and cervical vertebrae apparently suffered during a fall, perhaps while sleeping on the roof of his house, as was common then. A 30-year-old man was killed by a blow to his head. Osteoporosis (loss of bone mass in adults) has been found in a few mummies, but it occurred at earlier ages among the Egyptians than it does today among postmenopausal American women. X-ray studies of still other mummies have disclosed diagnoses similar to those seen in the royal patients in Cairo. All fail to reveal others that might have been expected, such as destructive cancers, rickets (because the Egyptians lived continually in the sunlight), and the few infectious diseases, such as syphilis, that can affect the bones (although there is both X-ray and dissection evidence of tuberculosis of the spine, which is probably always accompanied by infection in soft tissues).[38]

X-rays made in 1933 of five mummies at the Museum of Fine Arts, Boston, revealed little more, although the somewhat enlarged facial bones of one man suggest that he may have had acromegaly (abnormal bone growth caused by a hypersecretory tumor of the pituitary gland), a diagnosis found in a few other mummies.[39] Fifty years later, 11 mummies in the same collection, including some of those X-rayed earlier, were examined by both X-ray and computed tomography (CT), a technique that provides important technical advantages over radiography. The CT scans revealed more about the mummification process than about causes of death, but osteoporosis of the spine, accompanied by a fracture of the first sacral vertebra, and arteriosclerosis of a type suggestive of diabetes were found in the X-rays of a man who died about 930–880 B.C. (during Dynasty XXII). In addition, an elderly woman suffered from a molar abscess which went deep into her lower jaw, and one of her clavicles was broken.[40] CT scans of other mummies have shown an arrowhead in a Greco-Roman period man's mastoid process, and signs of pre-mortem healing around an apparent trephine wound in a Dynasty XVIII man's forehead. Other clear evidence of trephining (cutting a hole in the skull to relieve pressure from within, or perhaps to permit a demon to escape) in ancient Egypt is scanty at best, although six skulls from the Sudan and Sakkara, ranging in dates throughout Dynasties XIX–XXVI (about 1200–600 B.C.), appear to have such wounds; at least one was scraped out with a stone![41]

X-rays can reveal as much information about ancient teeth as about our own. The major dental finding among mummies is attrition, or extreme wearing of the crown, sometimes quite severe. It is found in as many as 93–100 percent of all jaws examined, including those of royal households from the Old to the New Kingdoms, as well as among modern Nubians. The Egyptians' teeth were continually worn down by the sand particles in their single most important dietary staple, bread, until, sometimes, no crowns extended beyond the bone surfaces of either jaw. In such cases, chewing was virtually impossible. No tooth decay at all was found in several series of ancient jaws, but caries was found in members of the court of Cheops, the Dynasty IV monarch who built the Great Pyramid, and in as many as 7.5 percent of all Egyptians who also showed bone loss around their dental roots. Caries, including several dental abscesses, has been detected in as few as 15 percent and as many as 33 percent of individuals in other studies; endodontal disease seems to have afflicted 80 percent of Dynasty IV and V Egyptians but only 12 percent in Dynasty XXV (712–657 B.C.). Similar correlations between chronology and incidence of caries suggest that it diminished in frequency over the centuries, although that conclusion is arguable. Attrition and caries could occur independently of each other, but the likelihood of developing caries increased as the teeth were ground further down, exposing the pulp to bacterial infection.[42] Egyptians who lived at various times down through the Middle Kingdom lost between 2.7 and 6.7 percent of their teeth.[43]

At least one specimen of a dislocated jaw has been reported; this was among the conditions a *swnw* might try to repair.[44] However, even if some Old Kingdom *swnw* did specialize in the teeth, it has been difficult to determine their therapeutic methods. Most dentistry probably involved only mouthwashes, although some of them were intended to be effective medications. The radiographic evidence, most of it negative and indirect, suggests that "toothists" did not open abscessed teeth. The oldest apparent example of prosthetic dentistry dates from Dynasty IV. It is a bridge made of artificially prepared natural teeth held together by a gold wire and attached to the abutting teeth. One other dates from 2000 years later.[45]

A few mummies have been "autopsied" to discover as much as possible about both the mummification process itself and underlying pathological changes. However, because dissecting a mummy is irrevocably destructive, it is seldom done. In addition, the specimens obtained may require unusual, elaborate, and expensive techniques for their analysis, far more than Drs. Granville and Pettigrew could ever have imagined. Even less encouraging, most published reports of mummy autopsies are disappointing in the extent of their positive findings. Many only duplicate radiographic observations, which require no destruction of the mummy itself. However, some autopsies have provided results that could have been obtained in no other way.[46]

For instance, several mummies have shown microscopic evidence of glomerulosclerosis (a deterioration of the vascular nests that filter urine from blood; it is usually initiated by a much earlier streptococcal infection, and may lead to hypertension), pericarditis (which could have produced heart failure), and cerebrovascular accidents ("strokes"). Noninfectious lung diseases included emphysema and pneumoconiosis (a pulmonary fibrotic disease associated with particulate contaminants in the environment). The ever-present desert sand was probably responsible for most cases of the latter, although many quarry workers and carvers were undoubtedly at even greater risk than the general population of ancient Egypt. In addition, carbon dust from exposure to wood fires in closed spaces was noted in two cases. Identifiable infectious diseases included both spinal and pulmonary tuberculosis (at least 31 cases of the latter have been reported), pleurisy, bronchopneumonia, mastoiditis, and osteomyelitis. There is some evidence that syphilis, leprosy, and small pox were present in ancient Egypt, but it is not unequivocal.[47] Periostitis (inflammation of the fibrous sheath of bones) has been noted in shin bones, but it was more likely to have been caused by insect bites than by trauma, which is probably the most common cause in modern America. Only a few benign and malignant tumors have been described, but none in the female breast; on the whole, cancers tend to occur at older ages than most Egyptians ever achieved. A few localized kidney diseases have been found, including an abscess and stones. A princess of the Middle Kingdom who had a vesicovaginal fistula died at childbirth because the infant was too large for her narrow pelvis.

There is considerable autopsy evidence for parasitic diseases along the banks of the Nile during all periods of Egyptian history, but little for malaria, which may have been a relatively late importation.[48] Among the parasites that have been positively identified in mummies are the dog tapeworm (*Echinococcus granulosus*, which causes hydatid disease), the pork tapeworm (*Taenia solium*, which usually produces only minimal symptoms), the guinea worm (*Dracunculus medinensis*, which migrates from the intestines to the skin and burrows out through it, causing debilitating pain in the legs), the large roundworm (*Ascaris lumbricoides*, which causes pulmonary and intestinal symptoms), the liver fluke (*Fasciola hepatica*, which causes gall bladder disease), threadworms (*Strongyloides stercoralis*, which also produces pulmonary and intestinal symptoms), trichinella (*Trichinella spiralis*, which causes fever and muscle pain if the larvae become encysted in muscle), and schistosomes (*Schistosoma haematobium*, which produce urinary difficulty and bleeding).

The finding of urinary tract stones in a few mummies raises the question of whether schistosomiasis (also called bilharziasis) was as widespread in pharaonic Egypt as it is today. The flukes that cause the potentially debilitating disease spend the reproductive portion of their life cycle in water snails of the genus *Bulinus*. We have no reason to suppose that schistosomes were first imported to the Nile Valley only recently, but they do find many more suitable breeding places there now that the Aswan High Dam no longer permits flood waters to flush the snails out to sea periodically; indeed, one-fifth of modern Egyptian deaths are attributed to schistosomiasis.

The flukes affect chiefly the softest tissues of the body, most of which were removed during mummification, so it is not surprising that stones, which can sometimes arise as a consequence of long-standing inflammatory reactions around flukes or their eggs, have been found only rarely, and in those few cases it may not have been schistosomes which actually caused the stones to form. Fluke eggs, which provide the best evidence of schistosomiasis infection in man, have been discovered in only a few mummies from rather late in ancient Egyptian history.[49] Several pictures of soldiers and workers have been said to show protective phallic sheaths designed to keep schistosomes from entering the urethra, but that speculative interpretation seems unlikely, since it would also imply that the Egyptians understood how the infection was transmitted. The time course of the associated symptomatology is such that it might have been quite difficult to make the connection between working in infested water and the characteristic symptoms of schistosomiasis, especially because it is not quickly or invariably fatal.[50]

The virtual absence of either textual or archaeological evidence for actual visitations of major epidemics of infectious diseases does not, of course, mean that none occurred. Even if none did, a spell to prevent "the Asiatic disease" in the Hearst Papyrus and eight incantations on the reverse of the Edwin Smith Papyrus (for which see Chapter Three) suggest that they were a source of continuing concern. All eight are spells for protecting the person who repeats them from afflictions such as "the pest of the year," or from another which comes "with the breath of every evil wind," while holding some appropriate magical object such as two vulture feathers. One spell is designed to remove, from the stomach and intestines, a fly which has been swallowed accidentally; however, it would be reading far too much between the lines to conclude from this that the Egyptians recognized that disease could be transmitted by flies.[51]

PUM II is the acronymically named (for Pennsylvania University Museum) mummy that has been subjected to the most thorough autopsy yet reported. The body was that of an uncircumcised male, 5 feet 4 inches tall (162 centimeters), who died about 170 B.C. (determined from both the style and radiocarbon dating of his linen wrappings) at the age of 35–40. The resins used in the embalming process had kept his body cavities sterile, although the remains of insects that breed in decayed flesh were found, trapped when preservative resins were poured onto the body. The fibrous covering of the right fibula was inflamed by an unknown cause. Several teeth were badly worn, and the jaws showed some associated resorption of their bony structure. The right ear drum had been perforated, perhaps purposefully, although it might have resulted from an infection. Only a small piece of the heart was found, but lipid plaques and fibrous arteriosclerosis were found in the aorta and other arteries. The lungs showed anthracosis, due to smoke, and silicosis, due to sand, although it could not be determined whether those pneumoconioses had caused respiratory symptoms during life. The spleen appeared normal, but the kidneys and bladder could not be found. The egg of a large roundworm (*Ascaris*) was found in the intestines. Histological studies revealed preserved collagen, the basic protein building block of the body, and even cell nuclei. Finally, it was found that PUM II had blood type B.[52]

Techniques other than destructive dissections or nondestructive radiography and CT scanning have revealed additional information about disease and death in ancient Egypt. For instance, studies of bones from

941 burials, from the Predynastic through the Christian eras, have hinted that malaria occurred along the Nile, but stronger proof is needed.[53] Techniques for detecting whether blood found on bones was shed before or after death were reported 80 years ago,[54] but they seem to have been neglected or abandoned since then. Visual inspection of bodies found in groups can reveal other kinds of information about ancient practices. For instance, most of 100 Nubians found in one place had been executed in Roman times by hanging, but the cervical vertebrae were intact, so their necks were not broken. Instead, the backs of their skulls were damaged in such a way that it could be concluded that their necks were virtually torn apart. A few other Nubian victims had been killed by decapitation, or by spears thrust into their loins or chest.[55]

The measurement of lead concentrations in teeth has provided good indirect evidence of changing methods for manufacturing metal objects, glazes, and paints. Because lead is a well-known hazard, such materials may have undermined the health of those Egyptians who have been found to have high dental lead concentrations.[56] For many years it has been assumed that the increased density and darkening found in the intervertebral discs of many mummies indicated disease, perhaps the exceedingly rare inherited metabolic disorder called ochronosis. However, new techniques, such as nuclear magnetic resonance studies, have shown that those disc changes occurred after death.[57] Other techniques that may permit adequate sampling of mummy tissues without doing significant damage to the body include biopsies taken through the body wall, and endoscopy, with instruments such as those now used to see into the living stomach, lungs, and large intestine, but these techniques require much more research before they are likely to become routine tools for Egyptological research.[58]

One of the most tantalizing mysteries of ancient Egyptian history, and of royal health on the banks of the Nile, surrounds the New Kingdom family of Akhenaten (or Amenophis IV, 1353–1335 B.C.) and Tutankhamun (1333–1323 B.C.).[59] In many, but not all, portrayals of Akhenaten, his face is elongated, and his habitus, including his abdomen and breasts, appears more feminine than masculine. Because his reign was characterized by a new sense of realism in Egyptian art, many scholars have tried to form a diagnosis based on images of him, and on his uncertain family tree. The suggested diagnoses have ranged from Vitamin D deficiency, to liver disease induced by schistosomiasis, to inherited hydrocephalus, to castration, to either acromegaly or Fröhlich's syndrome (also known as adiposogenital pituitarism), both of which can result from pituitary tumors, and on to others as well. Some of these would have been impossible in light of the fact that Akhenaten fathered six daughters—but in rebuttal it has been argued that they were not really his own biological offspring.

To further complicate the problem, some images of Akhenaten's father, Amenophis III (1391–1353 B.C.), Tutankhamun, and Smenkhkare, who reigned briefly between Akhenaten and Tutankhamun, show them, too, with gynecomastia (well-defined, though not fully formed, female breasts). Smenkhkare and Tutankhamun were full brothers, and probably full or half-brothers of Akhenaten, although we lack adequate evidence for proving all these hypothetical relationships. Thus, the last four kings of Dynasty XVIII may have shared genes that caused gynecomastia and even infertility—neither Smenkhkare nor Tutankhamun, although married for several years before they died, is known to have fathered any children. Or, the artists who portrayed them with various exaggerated features may have had their own reasons for doing so, some of which may as well have been rooted in religious symbolism as in a sense of realism. On the other hand, the men in the family may merely have inherited a peculiar body shape. We'll probably never know for sure.

3

SURGICAL PROBLEMS AND SOLUTIONS

Ancient Egyptian surgeons could provide practical solutions to problems whose causes were, by and large, nearly as self-evident then as they are today. Indeed, surgeons of all civilizations have differed from contemporary "internists" chiefly in their focus on localized rather than generalized conditions,[1] a dichotomy that persisted into the nineteenth century in the West.

There is no convincing evidence that *swnw* performed operative techniques that would now be classified as major surgery; most of it was relatively minor. For instance, Egyptian surgeons cauterized or lanced boils and abscesses, and they may have excised circumscribed swellings, such as wens and lipomas (fatty tumors). Several wall reliefs show anatomical protruberances that have suggested the presence of abdominal and inguinal hernias to some modern observers, although the pictures alone are not sufficient evidence for these diagnoses. A passage in the Ebers Papyrus hints not only that a *swnw* could demonstrate inguinal hernias by having the patient cough, but also that they could be reduced by manual pressure. Egyptian physicians almost certainly did not amputate limbs, but public executioners did perform punitive amputations of hands, nose, ears, tongue, phallus, and testes, and they even fractured offenders' arms and legs. In some cases the punishment was designed to fit the crime, as when the tongue was amputated for treason. Other penalties were less clearly analogous to Western punitive metaphors, such as amputations of the nose and ears of both adulterous women and corrupt judges. A much more common routine punishment seems to have been 100 blows with a staff and the infliction of five "open wounds" that would certainly have required treatment.[2]

We do not even know just what kinds of cutting tools Egyptian surgeons used for the operations they did perform, although blades struck from obsidian or flint were in general use by the early Old Kingdom. Not until the New Kingdom could small metal knives of appropriate shapes and sizes be made or imported, and even then such instruments were rare. Tools such as hooks, forceps, and "disposable" lancets and blades fashioned from reed stems have been inferred from procedures described in the medical papyri. The texts also allude to the "fire drill," which consisted of a stick and board used for starting fires by friction, as a cauterizing tool.[3]

Therapeutic bleeding is not mentioned in medical texts, although the papyri do note that snake and scorpion bites can be cured by sucking blood from the wound and applying a tourniquet around the affected limb. Even if bleeding had been a routine practice, venesection might have been difficult, since very sharply pointed knife blades were probably uncommon. Cutting edges struck from obsidian are quite sharp and might have permitted quick clean cuts.[4] However, as will be proposed later, the *swnw* probably had no good pathophysiological reasons for bleeding their patients.

The temple at Kom Ombo, built during the Roman occupation of Egypt and dedicated to the gods Sobek and Haroeris (also known as Horus the Elder), contains a celebrated enigma of Egyptian medicine. One wall displays a large relief (see Figure 10) depicting nearly 40 assorted instruments, including knives, spatulas or spoons, two or three small bags, vessels for holding liquids or oils, a pan scale similar to those customarily

FIGURE 10. The disputed "surgical instrument" relief on a wall of the temple of Kom Ombo. Several of the objects can be interpreted as knife blades, spoons (or spatulas), small bags for drugs (near the scales), and specula for dilating entrances to body cavities. In the lowest register, the two round objects are probably cups for bloodletting (introduced by the Greeks or Romans); the tall object next to them is a papyrus scroll; the bristly object cannot be identified even tentatively. Drawing by Yvonne Markowitz.

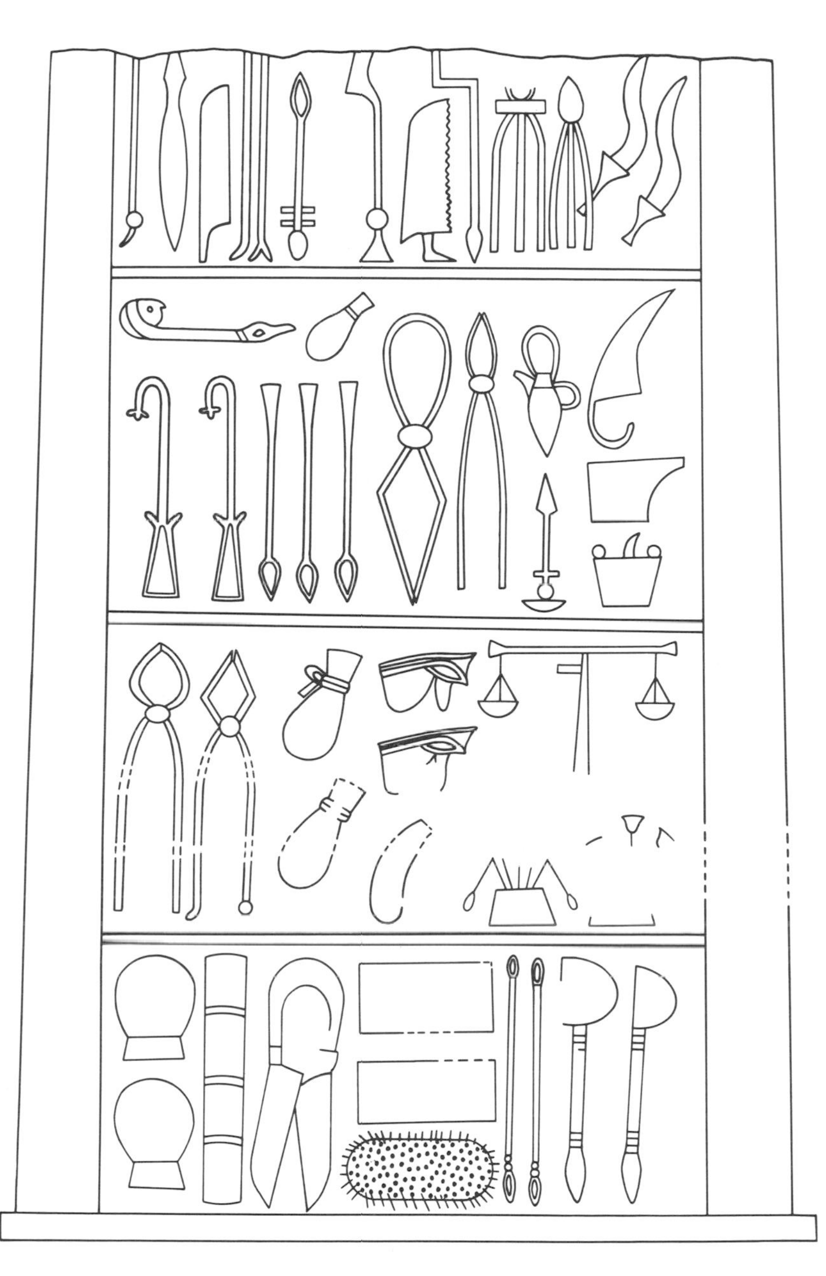

used for measuring drugs, and two stylized eyes of the falcon-headed god Horus (their special significance in medicine will be discussed later). Four objects may represent forceps, or even speculums for dilating and examining the cervix or rectum. The entire collection is being presented to Haroeris by the Roman emperor Trajan (98–117 A.D.) in his role as Pharaoh of Egypt.

Nearby inscriptions on the wall itself provide no clues to the objects shown in the relief; if there was an identifying inscription above, it was broken off long ago. An inscription elsewhere in the temple has been taken, on somewhat tenuous grounds, as evidence that these tools are for use in surgery.[5] One commentator considers them too large and clumsy for practical surgical use even if they are not drafted to the same scale, while others think that these objects were meant to represent goldsmiths' tools. Indeed, objects closely resembling those on the Kom Ombo wall can be found associated with many kinds of artisans in Egyptian wall paintings.[6] Nevertheless, virtually all the items are much like contemporary Greek and Roman surgical instruments.[7] Since there was a House of Life at Kom Ombo, it might not have been unreasonable to portray there a symbolic votive gift of standard tools of the surgical craft. However, because this relief is unique in Egyptian art, and because it is not clearly identified *in situ*, the problem must, technically, remain moot.[8]

Dentistry was already part of medical practice by Imhotep's time, when its practitioners, like Hesy-Rē (see Fig. 5), who were called "toothworkers" or, in one translation, "toothists," first appeared. However, the nature and extent of their practices, especially their operative techniques, are unknown. Neither mummies nor the medical papyri show conclusive evidence of invasive dental work. Radiolucent areas in a few mummy jaws have suggested borings performed to relieve bone abscesses, and one or two specimens hint that gold wire may have been used to keep single loose teeth from falling out, but the accumulated evidence is not strong enough to permit the conclusion that the "dentists" regularly employed either drilling or retentive techniques.[9]

Tooth crown wear caused by sand in the diet would not itself have required professional assistance, although it would have made chewing difficult. As noted earlier, the incidence of caries, which was uncommon in the Old Kingdom, seems to have increased over succeeding centuries; occasionally it resulted in alveolar (jaw) abscesses and even osteomyelitis, especially as the Egyptians' diet became sweeter and more varied. Most professional dental efforts seem to have focussed on drugs for inflammations and minor wounds of the lips and oral cavity, and for loose, and perhaps painful, teeth. That is, dental practice was more pharmacological than surgical.[10]

One surgical technique widely practiced in ancient Egypt, although not by the *swnw*, was circumcision. It was a ritual performed by priests, probably on large groups of adolescents or young men (but not infants). During the Old Kingdom only royalty, nobility, and priests were circumcised routinely. In later centuries the rite may have become obligatory for all pubertal males, perhaps as a precondition of marriage, but it may have been optional or even unavailable for some young men. Regardless of the extent to which circumcision was practiced, it seems to have grown out of the priests' concern for bodily cleanliness and, hence, purity, although it may have had some specific religious significance as well. Nor is it clear whether the operation involved complete removal of the foreskin or only its ritual nicking. Although several Dynasty VI statues (not all of them of royal personages) unequivocally portray complete removal, mummified remains are not very revealing; it appears that both techniques were used.[11]

The world's oldest portrayal of circumcision (Fig. 11)—in fact, the first known picture of any surgical technique—was carved on the wall of a Dynasty VI tomb about 250 years after Imhotep's death. The priest performing the ritual tells his assistant to hold the young man so he won't faint, and tries to make him comfortable. However, it was probably impossible to console a boy about to be circumcised with a stone knife. Afterward, honey and other emollients were applied to the wound to lesson the likelihood of bleeding and to speed the healing process.[12]

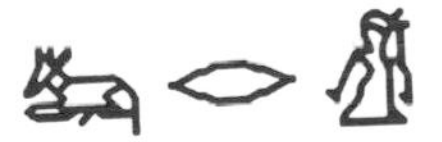

To become pregnant

Although gynecology and obstetrics are surgical specialties today, they involved no operative techniques in the ancient world. However, *swnw* did treat disorders of the reproductive tract, even during pregnancy.

The Egyptians recognized some of the procreative relationships among the testes, phallus, semen, and pregnancy. They regarded the man's contribution as a "seed" that he planted in the fertile ground provided by the uterus. Semen was seen as originating in the spinal cord (an association that persisted, on and off, into nineteenth-century Western medicine), probably because priests who made sacrifices thought that the phallus of the bull was an extension of his spine, since bovine *retractor penis* muscles arise from the lowest (sacral) vertebrae. The teleological importance of protecting the source of the man's semen by the large bone (which really represents the fusion of four or five vertebrae) at the end of the spinal column, coupled with its role in the myth of the dismemberment of Osiris, seems to have given rise to the bone's traditional name, the *os sacrum* ("sacred bone"). As far as more speculative Egyptians could tell, semen also arose in the heart, whence it passed via two pathways (called *metu*, to be discussed more fully in the next chapter) to the testes for later delivery into the woman. For instance, in describing the sex act, one text notes that the "man laid his heart in the woman." Although the maternal contribution to the fetus was not clear to the Egyptians, since they did not realize that sperm traveled to the uterus, nor did they recognize the ovaries, they did regard the mother's nutritional role, via the placenta, as vitally important.[13]

The exact duration of pregnancy may have been of little concern to the Egyptians until late in their history; the subject is virtually ignored in early texts. One text of unknown date specifies "up to the first day of the tenth month," while another mentions 294 days (9.8 months), simply because that was the length of the gestation of Horus, according to the prototypic national myth. The subject appears to have become more important, even if no better defined, when Roman law was imposed on the Egyptians. A ten-month gestation is mentioned in two texts from the Roman period that are concerned with the legitimacy of heirs, although one of these also specifies a lower limit of 182 days (six months). The

FIGURE 11. The circumcision scene in the Old Kingdom mastaba of Ankh-ma-hor at Sakkara, probably the oldest surviving portrayal of any activity even slightly surgical in nature. In the right-hand panel, the priest appears to be making the incision with a flint blade. The boy, who is probably pubertal, says, in the two vertical panels above him, "Obliterate really thoroughly!," and the operator replies, "I will make [it] agreeable!" In the left-hand panel, the circumcising priest, identified by the hieroglyphs in front of his head (but below the vertical lines), is probably applying a post-operative dressing. In the two narrow panels just above him, he says, "Hold him fast!" and "Don't let him swoon!" to the assistant who is holding the boy's hands out of the priest's way. The assistant replies, "I am doing to your satisfaction." Drawing by Yvonne Markowitz. The translation is from Alexander Badawy, *The Tomb of Nyhetep-Ptah at Giza and the Tomb of Ankhmahor at Saqqara* (Berkeley, Cal., 1978), 19.

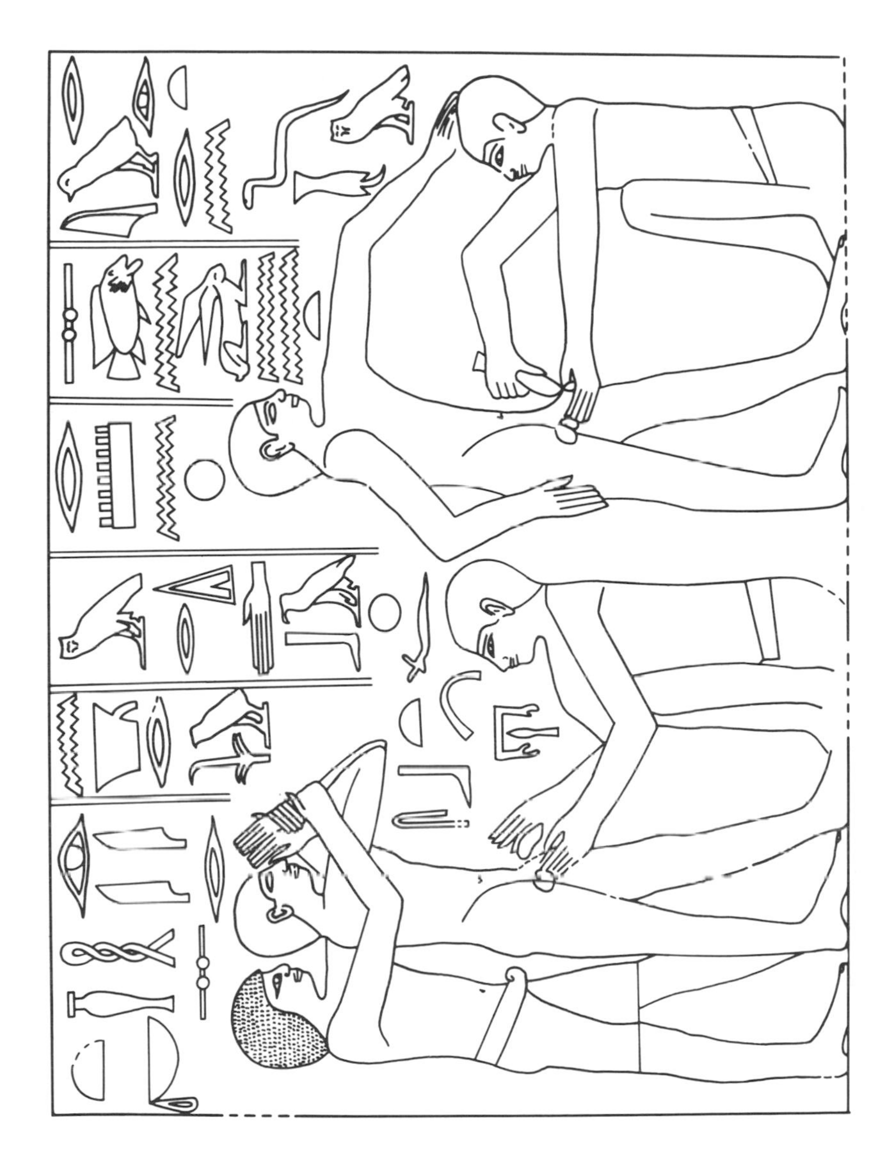

basic problem then, as well as earlier, was probably that no one knew how to determine the exact time of conception.[14]

Egyptians may have been more concerned with how to tell if a woman is pregnant. A number of chiefly magical methods for making the diagnosis have survived; none is predicated on the onset of amenorrhea (cessation of menses) as a clue. Several documents from both the Middle and New Kingdoms provide instructions for detecting whether a woman is capable of conceiving a child. One involves examining the "vessels" of her breast. Another states that the likelihood of becoming pregnant is proportional to the number of times the woman vomits while sitting on a floor that has been covered with the lees, or sediment, of beer and date mash. A third, also found in the much later Hippocratic writings, specifies that a woman can become pregnant if, on the day after an onion is inserted into her vagina, the onion's characteristic odor can be detected in her breath.[15]

But not all women wanted to become pregnant. The oldest of all the surviving medical papyri, the Kahun Gynecological Papyrus, which was compiled around 1900 B.C. during the Middle Kingdom, lists several recipes for contraceptives to be inserted into the vagina. They included pessaries made of honey with a pinch of natron, of crocodile dung in sour milk, of sour milk alone, or of acacia gum. Recently the latter has been recognized as spermatocidal in the presence of vaginal lactic acid, and it is conceivable that sour milk, too, might be an effective spermatocide.[16]

Predicting the sex of an unborn child was important to some Egyptians, and Berlin Papyrus No. 3038 (Dynasty XIX, about 1300 B.C.) gives one method for doing so: "Wheat and Spelt [a hardy wheat]: let the woman water them daily with her urine . . . in two bags. If they both grow, she will bear; if the wheat grows, it will be a boy; if the spelt grows, it will be a girl. If neither grows, she will not bear." The original rationale for this "test" probably lies in an ancient association of wheat and spelt with male and female divinities, respectively. In 1962 the method was assessed in a modern botany laboratory at Cairo, albeit in glass dishes rather than in bags. No germination was observed in samples treated with eight nonpregnant urines (including two from men), or in those treated with 12 of 40 urines from pregnant women; another five of the latter resulted in only poor growth. Statistical analysis of the raw data (chi-squared = 10.914, $P < 0.005$) suggests, as the recent investigators inferred, that the pregnant urine samples might have contained a substance that inhibited seed germination. However, the method provided correct predictions of the newborn's sex in only 19 of 40 cases, as would, of course, be expected on the basis of chance alone.[17]

In the absence of, or even despite, predictions about fertility or fetal sex, some Egyptians tried to exert direct influence on the outcome. For instance, milk from women who had been delivered of infant boys was given to a woman who wished to become pregnant, especially if she wanted a son. Mother's milk was sometimes stored for such use in jars shaped like a mother nursing her baby (see Figure 12), although human milk had several other nonspecific, and nonobstetric, uses in general "internal medicine."[18]

The medical papyri devote little attention to medical problems that might arise at the time of delivery, although the Ebers Papyrus suggests a number of oils, salts, and aromatic resins for hastening birth when inserted into the vagina, as well as two clearly magical procedures for preventing miscarriage. The same document also notes that if the baby says "*nj*" at birth, he will live; if he says "*mbj*," or moans, or turns his face downward, he will die. The mummy of one young woman shows that she died in or soon after childbirth about 1000 B.C., and another died because her infant's head was too large to pass between her pelvic bones,[19] but the overall incidence of perinatal deaths cannot even be guessed.

If all went well, when their time came women were delivered while squatting on two large bricks, or while sitting in a chair from which the center of the seat had been removed, as would become customary in medieval Europe. Women in labor were assisted, at least among the nobility, by two or three other women, not by *swnw*; New Kingdom pharaohs also knew that midwives and birth stools were employed by their Hebrew captives. Most of the few Egyptian pictures of birth show the infant emerging head first, as is normal. Indeed, the hieroglyphs for birth represent such cephalic presentations as well as the bricks.[20]

Although the *swnw* did not attend births, they did treat gynecological disorders, even if not with surgical techniques. They knew that amenorrhea and dysmenorrhea (absent and painful menses, respectively) were abnormal, and they administered a variety of soothing aromatic oils and ointments for inflammations of the internal and external genitalia. Many remedies for women's diseases are described in both the Ebers and Kahun papyri. The latter describes some ailments of the eyes, mouth, and legs, as well as those of the lower abdomen and the pubic area, as conditions resulting from "defluxions" (discharges, whether visible or not) of the uterus. The *swnw*'s concept of uterine anatomy was derived from the

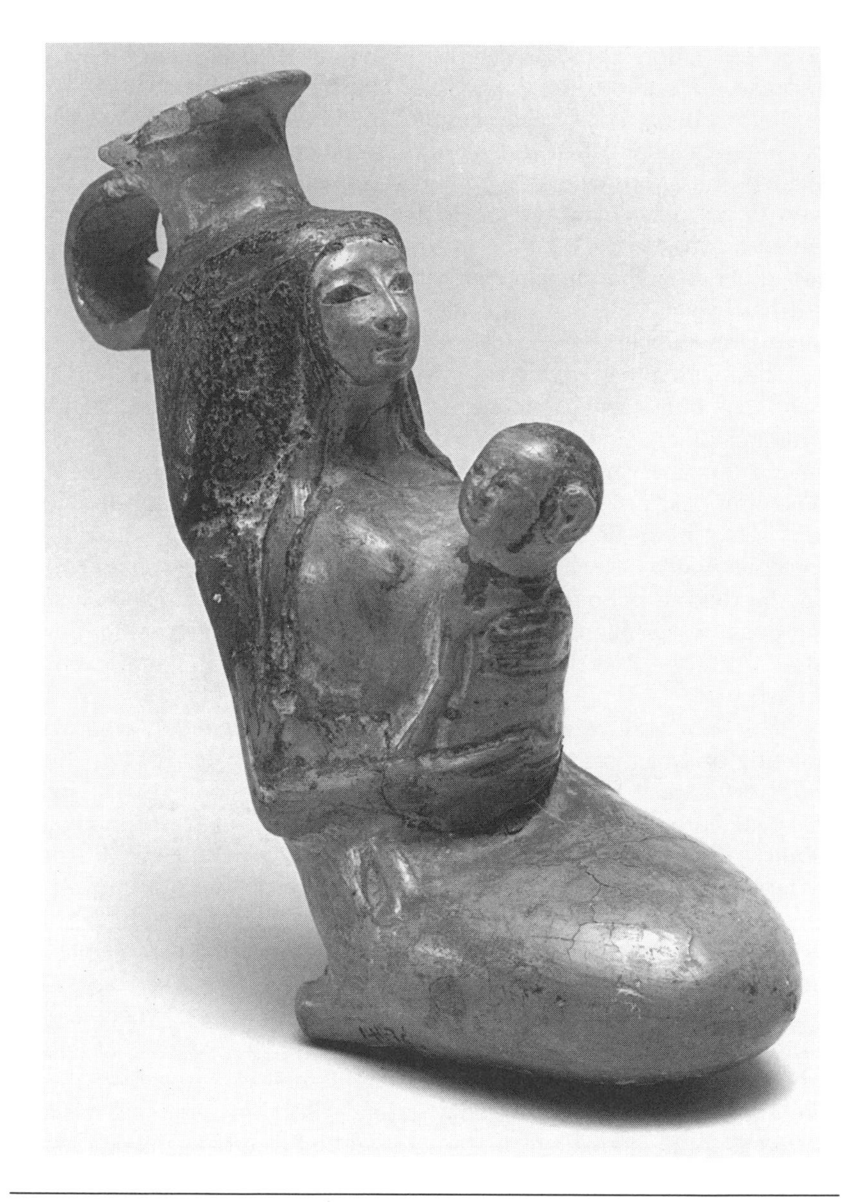

FIGURE 12. Red burnished ceramic bottle in the form of a woman and child, made about 1570-1293 B.C., and probably used as a container for milk for a woman who had a male child. (Courtesy of the Ägyptisches Museum, Berlin, 14476, Deibel Legacy, 1899).

bicornuate uterus of cows, which does not much resemble the single-chambered uterus of women. Because the *swnw* thought that many uterine disorders occurred when the womb became malpositioned in the abdomen, treatments for uterine symptoms relied largely on methods that physicians thought would force it back into its usual alignment, albeit with drugs, not by manipulation. Drugs intended to act directly on the uterus were administered by having the patient sit or stand over the burning ingredients, by directly inserting the remedies into the vagina, or by mouth.[21]

Wound

The Edwin Smith Papyrus, the "first edition" of which was probably written during the Old Kingdom, even if the surviving version was penned by a New Kingdom scribe, is the earliest document of major medical significance that has survived from pre-Hippocratic times. A compendium of 48 traumatic injury cases, the Smith Papyrus may have been intended as a reference text for a *swnw*, or perhaps simply as a student's copybook. Although the exact site of the document's discovery is not known, it may have been preserved in a physician's tomb for his use in the next life.

It contains the first written evidence of surgical procedures, and of deductive scientific reasoning (from observed facts to a clinical conclusion), and possibly (but very arguably) the first recognition that the brain controls certain motor and sensory functions, although the Egyptians did not build further on the clinical implications of those pioneering neurological observations. The manuscript even contains the first use of asterisks to indicate textual explanations and changes. John A. Wilson has noted that the content of the Smith Papyrus and the construction of the pyramids, among other achievements, permit us to eulogize the Old Kingdom as the period of Egypt's "highest intellectual achievement."[22]

The author of the Smith Papyrus carefully organized his cases by the anatomic sites of the injuries he describes, working down from the top of the skull to the facial and temporal regions, the neck, collar bones, upper arm, chest and ribs, and shoulders, and then to the upper spinal column, where the copyist unaccountably laid down his palette and reed pen, and stopped writing. The author also subclassified his cases systematically by the extent and severity of the injuries, and by their localization in bone, flesh, or both. Finally, he established a sensible procedure for dealing with each patient.

Examine, treat, or measure

His method begins with the physical examination, both visual and tactile; leads on to the diagnosis, based on facts elicited during the examination; and ends with a prognosis. The prognoses are of three standard kinds: treatable injuries; those of uncertain outcome that the physician will attempt to treat; and injuries, such as the most serious open or compound fractures, that are unlikely to respond to any treatment, although this last category also includes several minor conditions that required no treatment anyway. Because so many of the injuries described in the Smith Papyrus can be taken to be battle wounds or workplace injuries suffered at construction sites or mines, the unknown *swnw*'s prognoses can also be inferred to represent the earliest evidence of systematic triage, presaging Hippocrates' famous aphorism that "it is not enough for the physician to do what is necessary, but the patient and the attendants must do their part as well, and *circumstances must be favorable*" [emphasis added].[23]

The Smith Papyrus might well have been particularly useful to military surgeons. Fractured bones have been found in over 3 percent of about 6000 X-rayed mummies; most occurred post-mortem, during mummification or while the bodies were being forced into coffins that were too small for them. Of the rest, "many" were reported to have healed, especially fractures of the upper arm. However, the greater frequency of forearm fractures, compared to those of the upper arm, suggests that forearms were often broken during instinctive attempts to ward off blows aimed at the head. In battle, Egyptian soldiers had only hide shields and quilted helmets to protect them from the axes, maces, and throwing sticks that were among the favorite weapons of the time. Knives and swords were uncommon until late in Egyptian history, and bows and arrows, although standard weapons, would not have produced arm fractures. One commentator has suggested that the healed fractures permit us to infer that pus-forming bacteria were less common and less virulent in ancient Egypt than today, but neither this conclusion nor its underlying tacit assumption, that only modern antibiotics can halt infections, can be validated.[24]

The treatments recommended in the Smith Papyrus range from letting nature take its course, to cauterization, mechanical devices like splints, manipulative reductions of fractures and dislocations (even of the jaw), and medicines. Cauterization was applied with a fire-drill to a suppurating or very large tumor of the breast. Splints made of wood or linen rolls were used to immobilize fractured limbs, and the much later Hearst Papyrus calls for casts made of starches, such as barley flour, that would, when incorporated into bandages, harden like today's gypsum ($CaSO_4 \cdot 2H_2O$) or plaster-of-Paris ($CaSO_4 \cdot \frac{1}{2} H_2O$) casts. Wounds that penetrated the skin, such as those inflicted as punishments, as well as burns and bites (the latter more often inflicted by men than by animals), were to be treated by cleansing, drainage, and débridement (the surgical removal of injured or dead tissue); soap had not been invented. The most frequent topical remedy for wounds was fresh meat, to be applied only on the first day of treatment. Afterward, unguents composed of animal fat, honey, and copper ores such as malachite were usually applied. Another mineral included in many unguents has not yet been translated (it is transliterated as *imrw*). Only one case, a compound fracture of the frontal bone (forehead), includes an incantation as a remedy; although no prognosis was given, it may well have been considered predictably fatal. Adhesive gum plasters could have been used to hold wound edges together, and stitches may have been employed, but that is debatable (if so, it was the first time in recorded history).[25]

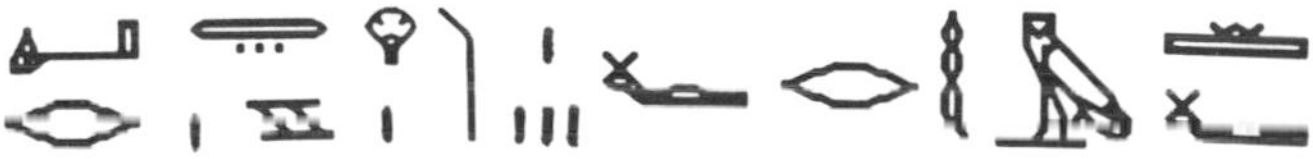

Moor him at his mooring stakes until he recovers

Other medical papyri also mention the two more favorable prognoses of the Smith Papyrus, but it is the only one that includes the verdict "an ailment not to be treated" (in 14 of 52 verdicts). Indeed, this prediction (as well as the other two) sometimes constitutes the entire diagnosis, and no specific treatment is mentioned. The papyrus also contains one other unique therapeutic recommendation, the injunction to "moor [the patient] at his mooring stakes." The metaphor of quietly mooring a boat at its home port on the Nile was already so archaic by the time this papyrus was written down that it had to be explained by the New Kingdom scribe as meaning "putting him on his customary diet without administering [any] drug." However, every time this procedure is recommended, it is accompanied by a *terminus ad quem*: until he recovers (one case), until the swelling is reduced (one case), until "you know he has reached a decisive point [e.g., a febrile crisis]" (one case), or until "the period of his injury passes by" (six cases).[26]

The Smith Papyrus—and Breasted's gradually unfolding commentary on it—reveals other "firsts" in the history of medicine. Some are moderately bizarre, such as the association of cervical vertebral dislocation with erection and ejaculation.[27] But most of the others reflect simply a common-sense approach to the diagnosis and treatment of wounds. Although many pages could be devoted to this document, it is undoubtedly most informative—and enjoyable—when read in Breasted's remarkably exciting—and scientific—exposition, a triumph of careful but colorful scholarship.

Egyptian physicians recognized that complete elimination of pus from wounds was an essential precondition to their successful closure and eventual healing. The belief that healing would be facilitated when all the disease-laden pus had escaped from the body may have given rise to the concept of "laudable pus" that survived into modern history. Some of the *swnw*'s conventional treatments for wounds would have permitted at least a modest amount of healing. The fresh meat applied to some wounds might have promoted blood clotting, but a *swnw* probably prescribed meat dressings because he had learned that "flesh mends flesh;" this may even have given rise to the use of steak for treating a "black eye" today. Because the *swnw* re-examined his patients after beginning their treatments, perhaps daily, in order to determine what further treatment, if any, was necessary, he had ample opportunities for evaluating the results of each therapeutic attempt at wound healing. In addition, merely changing the dressings on a regular basis would have been beneficial all by itself.[28]

A POSTSCRIPT FROM A MODERN LABORATORY

Although some of the *swnw*'s medications may well have provided effective protection from suppuration, he could not have understood that such medicines have antibacterial properties. Several inorganic salts prescribed by Egyptian physicians, such as those of antimony and arsenic, are now known to kill bacteria, but those of copper probably had an advantage over the others in that they were undoubtedly less toxic to the patient under the usual conditions of their clinical application in ancient Egypt.

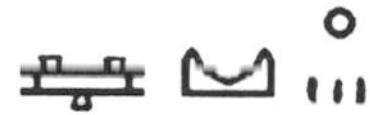

Green pigment

Copper salts, especially the bright green mineral malachite, were mined for decorative and cosmetic use in the pharaoh's court as early as about 2750 B.C., during the Old Kingdom. The author of the Smith Papyrus used what he called "a powdered green pigment" as a generic term for the copper ores he made into wound ointments. The major copper mines, in the Sinai peninsula, may have been opened during Zoser's reign. Reached by a trade route that led overland from the Nile through the desert valley of the Wadi Hammamat to the Red Sea, they were exploited throughout ancient Egyptian history, although their output increased during Dynasty XIX (1307–1196 B.C.), the time of Ramesses II. Copper compounds also came from Nubia, from Cyprus (its very name means copper) during the New Kingdom, and, just possibly, from the Near East beyond the Euphrates.[29]

Malachite is probably the active ingredient in 39 drug mixtures given in the Ebers Papyrus, which recommends it chiefly for afflictions around the eye and for open wounds, "to make the flesh grow." The author of the Kahun Gynecological Papyrus suggests applying it topically to what appears to be an infected swelling in a woman's groin. The author of the Smith Papyrus recommended "green pigment" for two purulent wounds, but the unusually systematic document breaks off before coming to what would probably have been a larger number of appropriate clinical indications for its use, if the Ebers and Kahun texts provide any clues.[30]

Guido Majno, a professor of pathology who has studied Egyptian wound treatments, pulverized samples of three ancient copper-containing materials in his laboratory and added them to bacterial cultures. Although he did not use different doses, his report leads to the inference that the salts' relative potencies were, from most to least active: verdegris (which contains cupric acetate), malachite (cupric carbonate), and chrysocolla (cupric silicate).[31]

A brief lesson in modern pharmacology can help explain some of the concepts I exploited in my own laboratory when I studied several ancient remedies, including the copper carbonate found in malachite. Pharmacology—the study of drug actions—compares drugs by focussing on their relative *selectivity, sensitivity*, and *potency*. If, say, an antibiotic kills off bacterial Species A at lower doses than are required to kill off Species B, the drug is said to be more "selective" for Species A than for Species B, while Species A can be said to be more "sensitive" to the antibiotic than Species B. Or, if a given dose of the drug kills off more individual bacteria of Species A than of Species B, the drug can still be said to be more "selective" for Species A than for Species B, and A is also more "sensitive" to the drug than B is.

Similarly, when we compare two drugs, if a species of bacteria is killed by smaller doses of Drug X than of Drug Y, we say that that species is more "sensitive" to Drug X than to Drug Y; we can come to the same conclusion if a given dose of Drug X kills more individuals of the same test species than does Drug Y. As a corollary, if Drug X exerts its effect, whatever that effect is, at lower doses than are required for Drug Y to produce the same effect, or if a given dose of Drug X produces a greater magnitude of effect than the same dose of Drug Y does, then Drug X is said to be more "potent" than Drug Y.

In my laboratory we used conventional modern pharmacological techniques to assess the relative selectivities and potencies of cupric sulfate (used today as a fungicide in fish tanks and swimming pools), cupric acetate, and cupric carbonate in cultures of the common infectious bacterial species *Staphylococcus aureus* and *Pseudomonas aeruginosa*. The experimental data (see Figure 13) show that cupric carbonate (found in malachite) is the most potent of the three salts tested, chiefly because it contains two copper ions per molecule of salt, while the other two salts contain only one cupric ion per molecule. Thus, when all three salts are equally solubilized, they are about equally potent in terms of their respective copper ion contents. We also found that all three copper salts are more selective for *S. aureus* than for *Ps. aeruginosa*, which is consistent with the greater complexity of the cell walls and membranes of Gram-

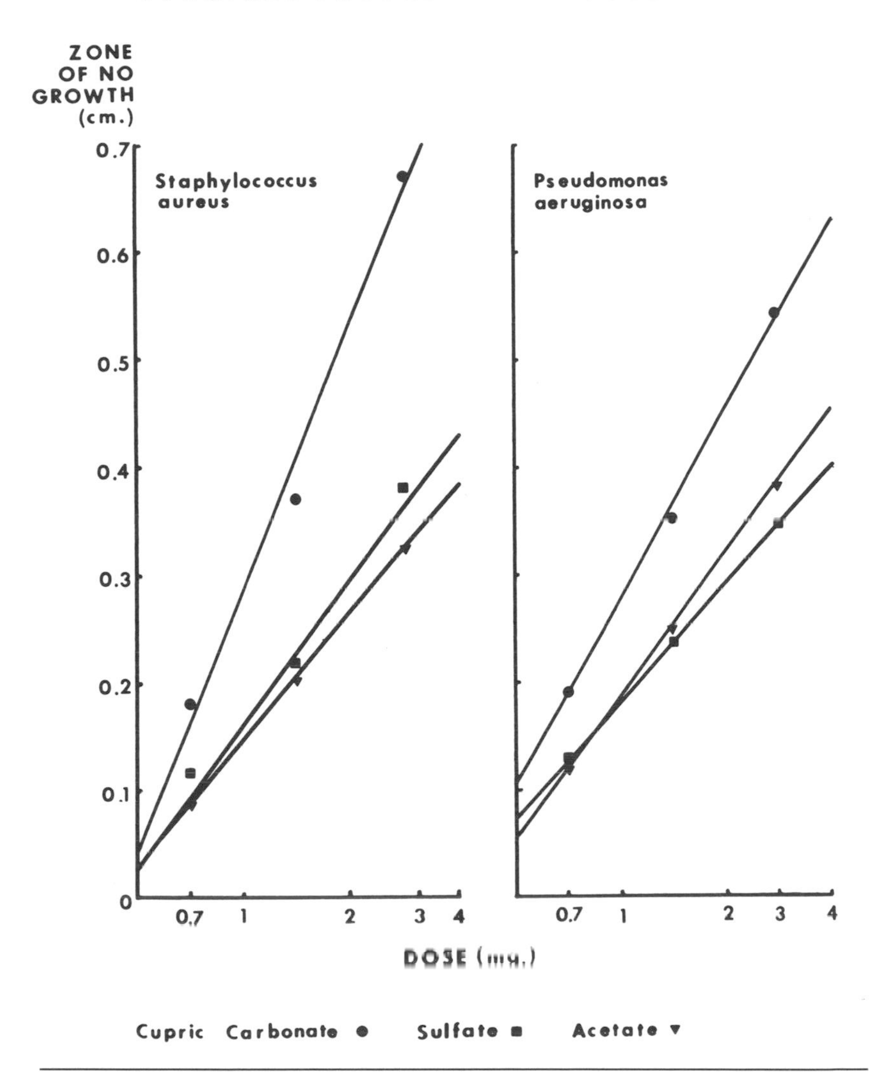

FIGURE 13. The effect of increasing doses of cupric carbonate, $CuCo_3 \cdot Cu(OH)_2 \cdot H_2O$, cupric sulfate, $CuSo_4 \cdot 5H_2O$, and cupric acetate, $Cu(CH_3COO)_2 \cdot H_2O$, in preventing growth of *Staphylococcus aureus* and *Pseudomonas aeruginosa* on agar plates maintained at 37°C for 24 hours. Because cupric carbonate achieves its effects at the lowest doses, it is the most potent of the three copper salts; cupric sulfate and cupric acetate are approximately equipotent in both bacterial species. Because the carbonate affects *S. aureus* at lower doses than those required to inhibit *Ps. aeruginosa* growth, the carbonate is concluded to be more selective for the former than for the latter; the other two salts are approximately equally selective for both organisms.

negative organisms like *Pseudomonas* when compared with those of Gram-positive organisms like *Staphylococcus*.

Thus, copper salts (the Egyptians, of course, used raw powdered ores, or greenish scrapings from copper pots and other vessels, not the purified chemicals we studied) might well have been therapeutically useful because, by inhibiting bacterial growth on open wounds, they would have allowed tissue repair to proceed normally. It was convenient for the ancient *swnw*, then, that *Staphylococcus* is more sensitive to copper salts than is *Pseudomonas*, because surface wounds are likely to become infected with *S. aureus*, while *Pseudomonas* is more likely to cause infection in the intestinal and urinary tracts. Consequently, we should not be too surprised that the Kahun Gynecological Papyrus recommends that women with what appears to be an infection in the pubic area should be treated with green eye paint boiled in cow's milk; the eye paint pigment was probably malachite, and the boiling would have facilitated solubilization of its chief ingredient, cupric carbonate. Nor should we be surprised that copper sulfate has been used as a home remedy for infections in the twentieth century.[32]

Although many plant products were recommended as wound dressings in the medical papyri, most are unlikely to have been therapeutically useful by today's standards. For instance, we found that a sample of myrrh from a local herb shop produced absolutely no antibacterial effect, even when we added large amounts of it to *S. aureus* cultures.[33] However, one indirect plant product—honey—looked more promising in the laboratory.

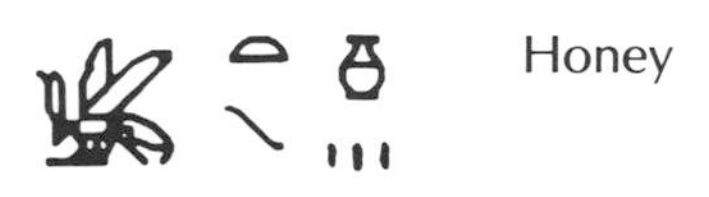

Honey

Honey was included in more ancient Egyptian medicines than any other ingredient presumed to have been therapeutically active. Although it was the most frequent ingredient in all the drug recipes for both internal and external use listed in the Ebers Papyrus and in the somewhat derivative Hearst Papyrus, it may have been intended largely as a pharmacologically inert diluent or vehicle in the oral medicines. Alternatively, its probable efficacy in many topical medications (such as those described in the Smith Papyrus) may have led to its eventual incorporation into oral remedies. The author of the Chester Beatty VI Papyrus (British Museum No. 10686), which is devoted entirely to disorders of the lower intestines, included it in nearly a third of the mixtures he recommended for administration directly into the rectum, even for treating disorders of far distant organs such as the heart; similar remedies are given in the Ebers Papyrus. However, since the *swnw* thought there were ducts that connected the anus directly to the heart or to surface wounds (see Chapter Four), the introduction of honey into the rectum presumably had a logical therapeutic rationale to ancient Egyptian physicians. Most important, the author of the Smith Papyrus directed that honey be applied topically, with few if any other possibly active ingredients, to more than half the wounds and sores he described. It is clearly the only presumably active ingredient in an ointment described in the Ebers Papyrus for application to the surgical wound inflicted in circumcision. Elsewhere that compendium specifies that an ointment for the ear be made of one-third honey and two-thirds oil (or perhaps animal fat). The concentration of honey in seven oral remedies in the Chester Beatty VI Papyrus ranges from 10 to 50 percent, while its proportion in five remedies administered directly into the rectum ranges from 20 to 84 percent.[34]

Beekeeping had been well developed by the Old Kingdom, and pictures of apiculture and honey processing survive from all periods of ancient Egyptian history.[35] However, the Egyptians could not have known that honey inhibits bacterial growth chiefly because it is hypertonic and, therefore, kills micro-organisms by drawing water out of them along an osmotic gradient. The bee's salivary glands also secrete the enzyme glucose oxidase, which favors the conversion of the glucose found in plant nectars to both gluconic acid, which is mildly antibacterial, and hydrogen peroxide, a common household antiseptic. Finally, bees collect, from nectars, a substance called propolis, which chemically resembles a modern food preservative, to repair cracks in their hives. Propolis was used by some eighteenth-century French physicians for treating skin infections, and it was marketed around the turn of the present century as a surgical antiseptic for postoperative use (under the trade name "Propolis hinvasogen"); reports from two surgical wards are said to have been favorable. Although propolis is no longer sold in the United States for medical use, as recently as 1973 an American physician reported that honey promotes the healing of burns and skin ulcers, and propolis is among the folk remedies available in modern Moscow. Majno has shown that the ancient mixture of one part honey to two parts animal fat can, in fact, inhibit the growth of *Staphylococcus aureus* and *Escherichia coli* cultures.[36]

To assess the relationship between dose of honey and its antibacterial effect, as we had done for the three copper salts, we added graduated doses of honey to broth cultures of *S. aureus* and hourly measured the increasing optical density produced by the growing numbers of bacterial cells, as shown for one representative experiment in Figure 14. All experiments showed a clear dose-effect relationship between the dose of honey added, up to 25 percent honey, and the magnitude of bacterial growth. When we added as much as 50 percent honey to the cultures,

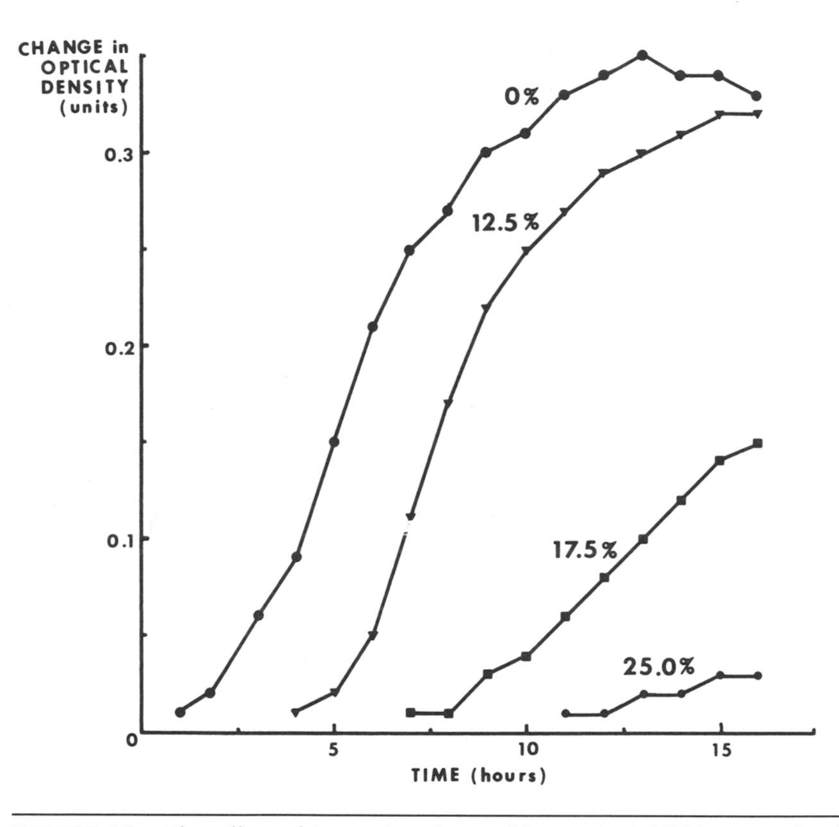

FIGURE 14. The effect of increasing doses of honey in inhibiting growth of *Staphylococcus aureus* in standard broth cultures maintained at 37°C for 16 hours. That honey can inhibit bacterial growth is demonstrated by the gradually decreasing transmission of light through the culture medium (when measured as optical density) as the dose of honey is increased. Solutions of 50 percent or more honey completely prevented any bacterial growth. See note 37 for further inferences based on the resulting dose-effect curves.

no growth at all occurred; thus, the ancient mixture that included 33 percent honey approximated the lowest maximally effective dose.

Honey's 80 percent sugar content accounts for its hypertonic properties. When we tested solutions of 80 percent glucose alone in the same way, we found that it, too, inhibits bacterial growth, although it is less potent than honey. This experiment confirmed that honey does, indeed, exert its antibacterial effect through other mechanisms in addition to its hypertonicity. We found that raw, unprocessed honey, freshly expressed from a comb, was more potent than bottled honey purchased in a grocery store. This is what we would expect to find because commercial honey is heated to 135° F during its processing, causing it to lose at least a portion of that part of its antibacterial activity that can be attributed to gluconic acid, hydrogen peroxide, and propolis.[37]

We could not bring ourselves to assess the efficacy of the Ebers Papyrus mixture of honey and oil (or animal fat). Nevertheless, the data we did collect strongly suggest that both pulverized copper ores and raw honey could well have provided some protection from the kinds of bacteria most likely to infect wounds, at least enough protection to permit the wounds to begin healing on their own. As a result, we are not very surprised that those ancient remedies from the banks of the Nile have occasionally resurfaced, even in modern times.

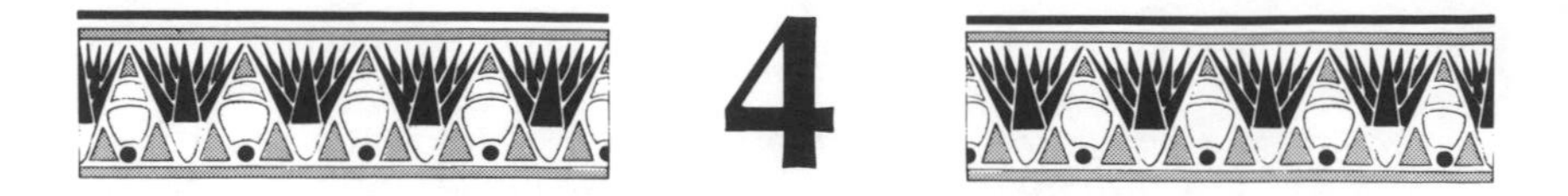

4

THE *SWNW* AND INTERNAL MEDICINE

The idea of health seems to have had positive connotations for the ancient Egyptians. To them it implied a sense of bodily vigor, not merely the absence of disease. The importance of health is evident in their everyday usage. For instance, the phrase "keep well" appears at the end of letters, and the word for health (probably pronounced *seneb*) appears in proper names such as one which translates "I am healthy."[1]

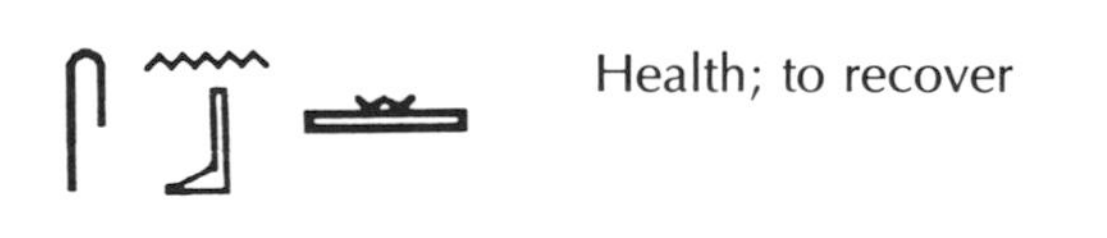

Health; to recover

Modern studies of ancient disease on the banks of the Nile have been summarized in Chapter Two. However, were it not for the medical and a few literary papyri, we would have little idea today of how the Egyptians themselves thought about illness from contemporary sources alone. Portrayals of disease are quite rare in their art, presumably because illness was considered inappropriate as subject matter for scenes to be "used" in the next life. On the other hand, sickness is nearly as rare in the art of later centuries, including our own.

A few diagnoses can be inferred from Egyptian funerary art, but it is likely that none of these ancient "patients" was symptomatically ill, at least in the minds of the artists who carved them. A Dynasty XVIII stele now in Copenhagen portrays a man whose right foot has been shortened in the past by poliomyelitis, or perhaps twisted by a congenital clubfoot abnormality called talipes equinus. Several reliefs and small statuettes represent men with severely curved spines (kyphosis), such as can be produced by Pott's disease, tuberculosis of the spine. Other sculptures show what is obviously achondroplastic dwarfism. Several reliefs have been said to portray conditions such as umbilical hernia and scrotal enlargement, perhaps due to tumor, as well as phallic enlargements, but they may also represent unskillful drawing or carving techniques.[2]

The prominent tortuous superficial arteries carved on the temples of elderly men suggest a diagnosis of advanced arteriosclerosis. Perhaps the most detailed and convincing Egyptian portrait of great age is a Dynasty XVIII relief in the Brooklyn Museum. It shows a man with wrinkled forehead and nasolabial folds, and sagging chins, and his collarbones and arm tendons stand out against the wasted muscles beneath them. However, he shows no signs of symptomatic illness.[3]

Nor are such signs evident among the numerous portrayals of middle-aged men with sagging waistlines; indeed, as noted earlier, some men wanted their statues to emphasize the rolls of abdominal fat that would advertise their well-deserved prosperity. But one truly startling case of obesity has survived, a famous relief that depicts Ati, the Queen of Punt, a country on the Somali coast that was visited by Egyptian trading expeditions. The relief, found at the funerary temple of Queen Hatshepsut (1473–1458 B. C.), shows that Ati suffered from a clearly pathological form of gross obesity. Her "case" was probably displayed in the Egyptian queen's temple because Ati was a distant foreigner whose portraiture required none of the conventions usually associated with those of native Egyptians, and perhaps because her obesity flattered the slender Hatshepsut.[4]

Pharaohs sometimes commemorated their military victories with vast reliefs that proclaimed their prowess on the battlefield and the fearful fates of their enemies, but there are few ancient pictures of the traumatic hazards of daily life in the home or workplace. One such has been found at Thebes in the New Kingdom tomb of an architect named Ipy. The precarious positions of the men building a large scaffold suggest they might fall off it at any time, while one workman actually drops a large hammer on the foot of another who immediately yells in pain. Elsewhere in the lively painting, a man, perhaps a *swnw*, appears to be reducing a workman's dislocated right shoulder, while another is applying what may be a medication to a laborer's eye. Above this last group is a small basketwork box typical of those used for drugs.[5]

First-hand evidence of disease is not much more frequent among nonmedical documents from ancient Egypt. In Dynasty VI someone writes to a deceased man, perhaps a relative, imploring him to "Heal your child! You must seize this demon and/or demoness now." In personal letters from the New Kingdom, a boy asks after his father's health, and a priest asks a colleague to pray for restoration of his health. A painter who has lost his sight asks his son to bring home three items frequently used in medicinal ointments: honey, fat or oil, and an eye paint, probably one made with malachite or stibium. Another man writes that he has "marasmus," which may mean that he is starved, although some wasting disease like cancer is also possible, and a woman reports that her servant is ill. Funerary steles tell how one man was blinded by the god Ptah, and how another died when a crocodile "sliced off" his legs. A third describes a woman whose breathing was paralyzed by a snake bite; however, she recovered after praying to the snake goddess whom she had offended. Another stele tells of a man who died within 24 hours of a scorpion bite, but there are many examples of such deaths, since snakes and scorpions were everyday hazards in ancient Egypt. Other documents mention men who had been legally punished with 100 blows. Many of these victims went into coma and died, but others survived, including an old man who was comatose for four days but recovered after three months of nursing care.[6]

A New Kingdom foreman at a Theban worksite recorded the reasons his men had to be furloughed. One had to take care of his sick mother; one was out for six weeks, perhaps because of a serious accident; and a third had been badly beaten in a fight with his wife. A man named Papet, who seems to have been a professional nurse or orderly, was assigned to take care of his fellow workers Apephti, Khons, and Haremouia, when they were sick.[7]

Longevity was a coveted mark of achievement. A courtier of Dynasty XXII (945–712 B.C.) was proud that he had "attained the age of ninety-six, being healthy, without illness."[8] A Dynasty VI text, "The Instruction of Ptahhotep," describes how an old man felt in his body:

Age is here, old age arrived,
Feebleness came, weakness grows,
[Childlike] one sleeps all day.
Eyes are dim, ears deaf,
Strength is waning through weariness,
The mouth, silenced, speaks not,
The heart, void, recalls not the past,
The bones ache throughout.
Good has become evil, all taste is gone,
What age does to people is evil in everything.
The nose, clogged, breathes not,
[Painful] are standing and sitting.[9]

This ancient writer had incurred many of the infirmities of age that are far more frequent today; they made him look forward to death as the resolution of his physical and mental problems. His despondency resembles the depression that still sometimes afflicts the elderly, especially when they have serious illnesses and psychiatrically significant depression. One can only assume that chronic geriatric illnesses also induced depression in ancient Egypt, while keeping in mind that few Egyptians lived long enough to develop them.

Several verses of a text now called "The Dispute between a Man and his *Ba*," written in Dynasty XII (1991–1783 B.C.) of the Middle Kingdom, provide a serenely hopeful view of death:

Death is before me today
[Like] a sick man's recovery,
Like going outdoors after confinement.

Death is before me today
Like the fragrance of myrrh,
Like sitting under sail on breeze day.

Death is before me today
Like the fragrance of lotus,
Like sitting on the shore of drunkenness.

Death is before me today
Like a well-trodden way,
Like a man's coming home from warfare.

Death is before me today
Like the clearing of the sky,
As when a man discovers what he ignored.

Death is before me today
Like a man's longing to see his home
When he has spent many years in captivity.[10]

Other sections of the "Dispute" might suggest that the speaker feels persecuted (one common refrain is "Lo, my name reeks") and isolated from others (another refrain is "To whom shall I speak today?"). Indeed, one interpreter was prompted to see the entire work as the "suicide note" of a man who was very severely depressed, perhaps even schizophrenic.[11] However, the translator quoted here is undoubtedly correct in her suggestion that the protagonist "does not appear to contemplate death as a suicide but rather as a natural, though greatly welcomed, death." The ancient author himself rejects premature, purposeful death as an acceptable solution to one's miseries, arguing that it should be left to fate alone to determine the time and manner of each man's death.[12]

Indeed, there is no direct evidence in any ancient Egyptian texts for severe psychiatric illness such as schizophrenia, partly because mental illness manifested as bizarre behavior could have been considered a supernatural phenomenon (e.g., a demoniac possession), partly because the Egyptians lacked any terminology for the psychiatric symptoms we recognize today, and partly because the schizophrenia syndrome was not recognized until early modern times.[13] Considering the modern view of schizophrenia as inherited, at least in part, it may have existed among the Egyptians, but there is no direct evidence that it did.

If the concept of health carried a positive connotation, and if death was seen as a natural end to life in this world, then the Egyptians' eminently practical view of how the various parts of their bodies functioned is not very surprising. The following nonmedical notions of human physiology stem from the belief that the ram-headed god Khnum makes each human body on his potter's wheel. Although the text dates from the Greco-Roman period (332 B.C.–395 A.D.), it surely represents ideas that had originated many centuries earlier:

He [i.e., Khnum] made hair sprout and tresses grow,
Fastened the skin over the limbs;
He built the skull, formed the cheeks,
To furnish shape to the image [i.e., the human figure].
He opened the eyes, hollowed the ears,
He made the body inhale air;
He formed the mouth for eating,
Made the [? throat] for swallowing.

He also formed the tongue to speak,
The jaws to open, the gullet to drink,
The throat to swallow and spit.
The spine to give support,
The testicles to [? move],
The [? arm] to act with vigor,
The rear [i.e., the anal area] to perform its task.
The gullet to devour,
Hands and fingers to do their work,
The heart to lead.
The loins to support the phallus
In the act of begetting.
The frontal organs to consume things,
The rear to aerate the entrails [i.e., at defecation],
Likewise to sit at ease,
And sustain the entrails [i.e., prevent defecation] at night.
The male member to beget,
The womb to conceive,
And increase generations in Egypt.
The bladder to make water,
The virile member to eject
When it swells between the thighs.
The shins to step,
The legs to tread,
The bones doing their task,
By the will of his heart [because it was thought to be the seat of the mind].[14]

Thus, not only was the Egyptian able to recognize many basic correlations between structure and function, he had opportunities, such as this prayer, to hear them, see them, or repeat them. That is, these rather obvious physiological concepts were not just vague notions floating loosely around in ancient thought; they were reinforced in texts like this one. However, since the human body had been designed and given concrete form by a god, even if not precisely in the god's own image, both health and disease could also be interpreted within a supernatural context, and not solely on the basis of empirical, much less "scientific," observations.

The *swnw* who specialized in "internal medicine" had to go much further in his understanding of disease. He was no less rational or empirical than his surgical colleagues who practiced "external medicine," but the underlying causes of the clinical problems that confronted the ancient "internist" were less visible to him. He might conclude that injuries, and even some internal symptoms, were caused by accidents, or occasionally by enemies or malevolent fiends, but he could not interpret all nontraumatic illness in terms of such self-evident cause-effect relationships. Because he could not—or at least did not—test his theories of how the healthy body works, the *swnw* developed an equally untested concept of the pathological basis of disease. Nevertheless, upon this speculative interpretation of his observations he developed a logical therapeutic system.[15]

Steuer and Saunders have postulated that, "Throughout the history of medicine the physician has searched for a theory of disease through which he might organize a diversity of data and justify his practice by establishing a scientific system. . . . Since the fundamental problems of disease remain the same, initial hypotheses tend to persist and early ideas in medicine, modified in some form or other, have a habit of making their reappearance from time to time."[16] Ancient Egyptian medical hypotheses were extraordinarily long-lived, partly because the *swnw*'s empirical observations satisfied him that his theory was not fallible, and partly because his religious beliefs anthropomorphized and synthesized many observable laws of nature. This permitted the "internist" to rely on unprovable theory, and even on magic, more than the "surgeon" found necessary.[17]

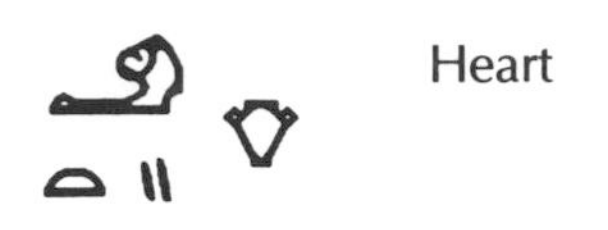

Heart

Henry Sigerist carried the explanation of primordial medical systems another step further when he concluded that "Physiology began when man . . . tried to correlate the action of food, air, and blood."[18] The Egyptians found the focal point of this correlation in the heart, which they regarded as the central organ of the body, essential to both the living and the dead. They reasoned that all the senses report directly to the heart, that it was the seat of thought, emotion, and intelligence. Lacking a word for "mind," they used "heart" to represent the same idea. It was, therefore, the seat of life as well as of both good and evil thought—of the conscience. This, in turn, required that in the netherworld the heart of the dead was to be compared, on pan scales, with a feather: the deceased was permitted to progress in the afterlife only if his heart, representing his conscience, did not weigh more than the feather representing law, truth, and order (*ma'at*). (Virtually everyone seems to have passed this test). Because the deceased would need to have his heart available for weighing in the Hall of Judgment, embalmers left only it, among the major organs they knew, inside mummies (although in late Egyptian history they often substituted artificial representations of it).[19]

Most of what we know about the Egyptians' physiological concepts comes from the Ebers Papyrus. Although the manuscript dates from the New Kingdom, the steadfast conservatism of ancient Egyptians, their

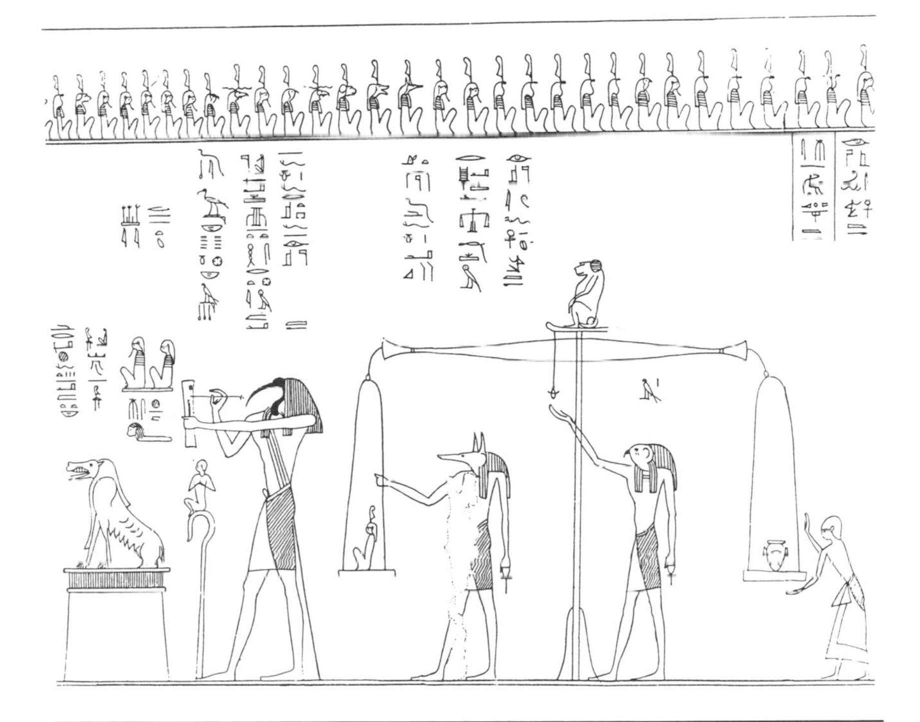

FIGURE 15. Weighing the heart in the netherworld, from a twelfth-century B.C. papyrus. The heart is on the right-hand scale; a figure of Ma'at, symbolizing truth and wearing the symbolic feather, sits on the left. The ibis-headed divine scribe Thoth stands to the left of the scale, writing down the results of the weighing; in the unlikely event that they are unfavorable, the deceased will be devoured by the monster sitting on the pedestal to the far left. A baboon, sacred to Thoth, sits on the balance post of the scales. From Richard Lepsius, *Das Todtenbuch der Ägypter nach dem Hieroglyphischen Papyrus in Turin* (Leipzig, 1842).

inability to test their physiological ideas, and several textual clues, suggest that many if not all of the same theories had originated by the Old Kingdom. Indeed, part of the Ebers Papyrus seems to have been taken from the same source as the section of the Smith Papyrus called *The Physician's Secret: Knowledge of the Heart's Movement and Knowledge of the Heart*. Although some interpreters differ slightly in their translations and conclusions, a general outline of the *swnw*'s physiological theories can be ascertained in the Ebers document (as well as in similar sections of the Smith and Berlin No. 3038 papyri).[20]

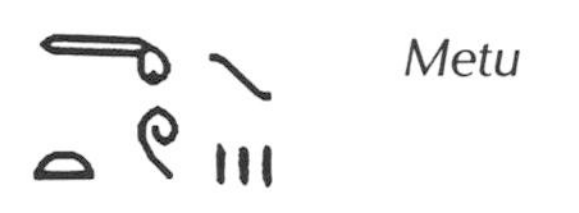

Metu

The *swnw* regarded air as vital to life and to each organ of the body. It entered the body through the nose and traveled through the trachea directly into the heart. Air left the heart in the blood, along with water, which was also essential to life. Together they traveled via a series of afferent ducts called *metu* to each of the body's organs. From some of the organs a second set of efferent *metu* carried those organs' respective products or excrements to the surface, as seen in Table 1. (Note that sweat is not among the products of the secondary *metu*, presumably because under normal desert conditions it evaporates so rapidly as to be virtually imperceptible.)

The medical papyri differ somewhat in the exact number of *metu* that they ascribe to each area of the body, and in the total number listed by each text, but the various descriptions are not necessarily mutually exclusive. Moreover, the differences were of little practical significance to the *swnw*, nor should they be to us; since the *swnw* could not differentiate among arteries, veins, nerves, and tendons, he lumped them all together as *metu*. If the author of the early *Physican's Secret* had never read any other medical texts, his own "counts" would be just as valid as those of later authors.

Thus, the Egyptians considered the *metu* to be indispensable to normal body function, inasmuch as they were the principal means for transporting blood, air, and water to nourish the various organs. The importance of healthy *metu* even to nonphysicians is implicit in everyday ancient wishes such as "may his *metu* be comfortable," and in greetings such as "may thy *metu* be sound."[21]

TABLE 1. The basic *metu* system, according to the Ebers Papyrus. Variants of this overall plan are also included in both the Smith and Ebers papyri.

AIR (via the Trachea) and
WATER (via the Stomach)

enter the *HEART* from which, along with *BLOOD*, they are sent, via *PRIMARY [AFFERENT] METU*, to the

LOWER INTESTINAL TRACT [4 *metu*][1]
STOMACH or BELLY [? *metu*]
LUNGS and SPLEEN [4 *metu*, probably 2 to each][2]
LIVER [4 *metu*][2]
LIMBS [3 *metu* to each, extending as far as the fingers and toes]
BUTTOCKS or THIGHS [2 *metu*]
EARS [2 *metu* to each][3]
FOREHEAD [2 *metu*]

	PRODUCTS OF SECONDARY [EFFERENT] METU
TOP OF HEAD [2 or 4 *metu*]	Baldness
NOSE: 2 *metu* secrete:	Mucus
2 other *metu* secrete:	Blood
EYES [2 *metu* each]	Tears, through pupils
TESTES [2 *metu*]	Semen[4]
BLADDER [2 *metu*]	Urine[5]

1. These afferent *metu* of the lower intestines can also transport *wḫdw* (and undigested food residues) backward, i.e., to the heart.
2. Disease arises in these organs when they overflow with blood.
3. In addition, the Ebers Papyrus states that the breath of life enters the right ear, while the breath of death enters the left ear.
4. Its active principle was thought to arise in the spinal marrow.
5. The kidneys and ureters, and their relationship to the bladder, seem to have been completely unknown to the *swnw*.

Although this highly speculative physiological system was not based on sound anatomical or experimental observations, it led to a general model of disease that seems plausible enough if you can accept the existence of *metu*—which was not difficult to do 4500 years ago. The *swnw* believed that imbalances of air, water, and blood within the *metu* were disseminated throughout the body, or to its surface, depending on which, and how many, *metu* were affected. For instance, it was to assess the condition of specific *metu* that a physician would palpate his patient's pulse in the head, neck, arm, groin, or leg. The most important cause of disordered *metu* was a substance that is commonly transliterated as *wḫdw* (and pronounced something like *ukhedu*), which has been characterized as "the rotten stuff par excellence." Its travels through the *metu* are described in the section of the Ebers Papyrus titled *The Collection on Expelling the Wḫdw*. Like the *Physician's Secret*, the *Collection* was copied from an earlier text said to have been composed during the reign of Usaphais (also called Den) in the First Dynasty.[22]

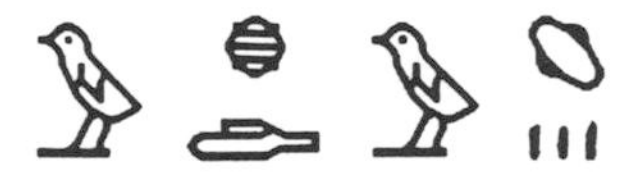

Wḫdw

Just as decay and foul odor characterize death, so are they associated with the feces of the living. *Wḫdw* originated in the feces, thought the *swnw*, as residues of undigested food, and it is, of course, in the large intestine that post-mortem putrefaction begins or is most noticeable. If, then, *wḫdw* were allowed to accumulate to a dangerous level within the rectum, the pathogenic *wḫdw* would overflow into its afferent *metu* and travel backward to the heart, whence it could then be distributed, via other afferent *metu*, to the several organs. The Egyptians even explained the proliferation of disease—or, more accurately, symptoms—in old age by assuming that more *wḫdw* was absorbed from the intestines by the *metu* of the elderly than from those of the young.

Although *wḫdw* was usually considered to arise in the feces, it might also appear in open wounds, and both of these fountainheads could activated by magic as well as by disease or injury. However it originated and spread, *wḫdw* was thought to be converted to pus after it had entered the blood within afferent *metu*. Then, when it settled into a target organ, putrefaction would set in. Finally, the pus coagulated the blood, which is, of course, the mark of initial healing of a wound, as the scab. The Egyptians used the term "Blood-Eater" to describe the *wḫdw*'s ability to change the blood and cause disease, inasmuch as the clot was interpreted as the final destructive result. Thus, the surgical *swnw* might try to prevent scab formation over a wound, so that pathogenic *wḫdw* could escape from the body. Among the terrifying demons in the Hall of Judgment, before whom the deceased had to declare himself innocent of specified sins, were a "Blood-Eater" and an "Eater-of-Intestines," who probably represented related fears of corporeal corruption.[23] Thus, although the word *wḫdw* does not appear in the Smith Papyrus, it was surely part of the "surgical" reasoning expressed in it.

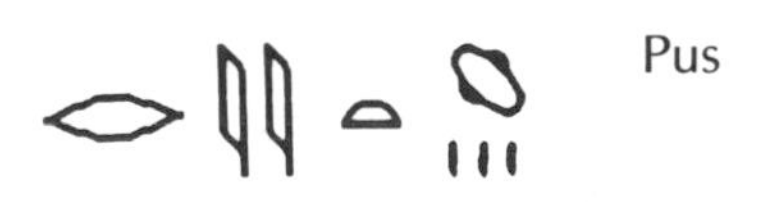

Pus

The *wḫdw*, which came in both male and female forms, could itself be killed. Therefore, just as the putrefaction of death was conquered with natron in the mummification workshop, so further accumulation of the putrefying *wḫdw* was to be prevented in the living with measures such as washing, styptics, wound ointments, emetics, cathartics (around which much of the ancient Egyptian's medicinal effort revolved, as we will see), and lancing of purulent accumulations such as boils. The same word was used to mean "to embalm" in the Book of the Dead and "treatment" in the medical papyri, although the words referring to mummification in the Book of the Dead lack the determinative hieroglyphs pertaining to corruptibility that were used with the word *wḫdw*.[24] It was probably axiomatic to the *swnw* that wounds could not heal completely until all pus had been eliminated from them. Bleeding might have been a logical method for removing *wḫdw* from the body, but it was not regularly exploited as a therapeutic measure before Greek culture was introduced late in ancient Egyptian history.[25] Perhaps most *swnw* reasoned that loss of blood and its vital contents would be more hazardous (and less effective as a primary treatment) than prophylactically accelerating the escape of *wḫdw* from its site of origin in the intestines.

Overindulgence in food and drink was considered potentially unhealthy because the excessive residues that they would leave in the gastrointestinal tract would facilitate the development of *wḫdw*. Several injunctions against gluttony are found in the morality literature. Although the surviving texts date from Greco-Roman times, their message is far more ancient:

> *Illness befalls a man because the food harms him.*
> *He who eats too much bread will suffer illness.*
> *He who drinks too much wine lies down in a stupor.*
> *All kinds of ailments are in the limbs because of overeating.*

He who is moderate in his manner of life, his flesh is not disturbed.
Illness does not burn him who is moderate in food.[26]

As noted earlier, some foods were considered taboo, not because of any now recognizable pathogenic micro-organisms they might have harbored, but because eating them would offend the god with whom they were associated and prompt him to retaliate against the offender by producing *wḫdw*. The winds, especially when stronger than usual, or when blowing from uncommon directions (usually they came from the north), were sometimes said to bring poisonous materials; so could demons, such as the "pest of the year," or even the spirits of the dead.

The only readily visible, presumably pathogenic factors in ancient Egypt were worms and insects; they could actually be seen to aggregate on suppurating wounds or occasionally around the eyes or anus. However, it probably did not occur to the *swnw* that such infestations were more likely to be secondary rather than primary instruments of disease. And, if real worms were associated with such problems, then some symptoms could be interpreted as having been produced by rather metaphoric or hypothetical worms, especially the still unidentified *āaā* disease (which appears, contrary to early opinions, not to have been either hookworms or schistosomes). If none of all the known causes of illness could be invoked for a patient, his *swnw* could conclude that the illness at hand was attributable to an occult cause, such as a demon or a god's vengeance, or to a "moral cause" like homesickness, love, adultery, or homosexuality. Moreover, even demoniac or moral causes of disease could be transmuted into physiological causes, such as *wḫdw*.[27] In any event, ancient Egyptians seem to have had little sense of symptom causation beyond what an observer might have thought happened just before, or during, the phenomenon for which a cause was sought.

Perhaps Egyptian notions of disease and its origins would not be so elusive today if more documented evidence of epidemics and their effects on the population were available. As it is, there is virtually none; nor is there convincing evidence that the Egyptians had even the most rudimentary concept of contagion.[28] Even the formulas for exorcising the "pest of the year" on the reverse of the Smith Papyrus[29] provide no helpful identifying clues to annually recurring epidemics that could be transmitted to or among the dwellers on the Nile.

Cleanliness was an everyday concern, perhaps even a preoccupation, of Egyptians of all classes, but there is no evidence that it was fostered by fear of contagion. Bathing areas, in which water was poured over the bather while he stood or squatted on a stone slab with raised edges, have been found in private and royal homes. Beards and other body hair were regularly removed, especially by priests, who also shaved their heads. They probably used oils or unguents as softening agents because they had no soap. (Actually, embalmers made soap every time their natron mixed with the triglycerides in animal fats, a reaction that produces glycerol, carbon dioxide, and the sodium salts of fatty acids, which are among the soaps. However, the Egyptians seem not to have separated out their soaps and discovered their cleansing properties.) Some softening was needed, since the poor had to use flint knives or scrapers for shaving, although reasonably sharp copper or bronze razors were available to well-to-do men and women.[30] Religious or ritualistic demands may have underlain the practice, but it is tempting to speculate that shaving might also have permitted free exit of *wḫdw* from those *metu* that terminated in the skin or hair.

In addition, the Egyptians had to dispose of their urine and feces, especially because they were so closely associated with disorders of the *metu*. Most villagers probably relieved themselves in fields or other convenient places, but some houses had latrines. One was built in a Dynasty II (2770–2649 B.C.) tomb (no. 2302) at Sakkara. It consisted of a dish half filled with sand and placed below a rectangular hole cut into the seat, which rested on bricks that fanned out as they rose from the floor. Although a privy might seem inappropriate for a tomb, it can also be seen as a logical necessity inasmuch as the deceased was plentifully supplied with food for his next life. Latrines have been found in the remains of a royal palace built about 1180 B.C., as well as in the houses of high officials and even lesser homes at Tell el-Amarna (e.g., houses 0.48.1, 0.48.4, T.36.11, and T.36.36). Portable wooden stools, with keyhole shaped holes cut into the seats, were also used indoors. Drains and copper pipes for removing sacrificial wastes have been found at a Dynasty V (2465–2323 B.C.) temple at Sakkara, but the system was not very satisfactory, and it was not used elsewhere. Moreover, there is no evidence that such constructions were used as outlets for domestic lavatories. Latrine pots were emptied out of doors, perhaps in a designated communal refuse heap; several areas that probably served that purpose have been excavated at Tell el-Amarna. Similarly, water used for bathing was collected in subsurface pots for later disposal, to keep bathroom floors dry. The Egyptians relied on the scorching sun to evaporate their fluid wastes; they could not have known about microbial contaminants, of course, but the desiccating heat would have killed most of them.[31]

The actual extent to which the *swnw* thought about the *wḫdw* in his day-to-day work cannot be determined, but both he and the population at large appear to have been preoccupied with keeping the intestines free of the one major "pathogen" they knew. To accomplish this goal, Egyptians took cathartics at regular intervals, so that unhealthy amounts of *wh̆dw* could not accumulate. This prophylactic habit was so widespread, and indulged so frequently—three days each month—that in the fifth century B.C. the Greek historian Herodotus noted it with amazement.[32] It will be seen later that the *swnw* differentiated between disease of the *metu* and other, more magical, kinds of intestinal disorder, but the two categories may not have been mutually exclusive.

Anus, or lower intestines

The Egyptians' concern with the anus, the terminus of the intestinal tract and the optimum primary drainage site for *wh̆dw*, is also reflected in their surviving drug prescriptions that are concerned with anal conditions. All the papyri describe conditions such as "hot anus," "warm anus," rectal prolapse (or falling out of place, whether real, through the anus, or presumed, as in the uterine "defluxions" mentioned in Chapter Three), and, probably, ordinary hemorrhoids. (We will continue to use the translation "anus" here, although the word transliterated as *pḥwy* really referred to the entire alimentary tract below the stomach.[33]) The hieroglyphic word for medicines (transliterated as *pẖrt* and probably pronounced something like *peckeret*), included both the symbol for pills and that for the intestines, which seems to reinforce the association even more. Perhaps the Egyptians devoted so much attention to the anus because clear-cut symptoms such as diarrhea are hallmarks of the gastrointestinal diseases that probably were common then. However, more of the Egyptians' medicines were designed to move the bowels, and were presumably effective (insofar as they could tell) for the job, than were used to control diarrhea. This suggests that natural evacuation of the *wh̆dw*, even as diarrhea, was regarded as desirable, and that drugs were thought to be most useful when the noxious material could not be passed out of the body by the normal fecal route.

It is difficult—if not impossible—to reconstruct the full range of the *swnw*'s diagnostic criteria and skills from the papyri. Many descriptions of nontraumatic illnesses are sketchy, at best, opening wide the gates of overenthusiastic temptation to make them fit modern medical terminology. Moreover, we still lack English equivalents for many critical hieroglyphic words, precluding even carefully measured attempts to read modern concepts between some of the pictographic lines. Nevertheless, the medical papyri, taken in conjunction with information gathered from mummies, do permit us to compile a tentative outline of the damage that absorbed excesses of *wḫdw* could do, insofar as the *swnw* could tell.[34]

No "Manual for Examining Patients" has survived from ancient Egypt. The directions sporadically given in the medical papyri permit us to form some idea of what the *swnw* might do and look for when he encountered a new patient, even if he was not as uniformly systematic in his examinations as modern physicians are trained to be. Even if he began by asking the patient what the problem was, there is little evidence that the *swnw* routinely asked about specific details of the patient's medical history. The physician might note his patient's general appearance, skin color, and nutritional status, as well as his state of consciousness and his memory ("perishing of the mind"). He might evaluate secretions from the nose, eyes, and ears, and try to detect the unmistakable odor of corruption in the sweat, breath, and wounds. The *swnw* also noted whether the patient was shaking, and looked for what we now recognize as swollen varicose veins.

Finally, if indicated by the nature of the patient's chief complaint, he palpated the abdomen, including the inguinal and scrotal areas (to detect hernias and perhaps tumors), and felt for fractures, dislocated joints, and, probably above all, the pulses of the wrist, foot, stomach, groin, head (perhaps the temples), and the neck. Indeed, the author of the Smith Papyrus regarded the motion of the heart, palpated in any of the peripheral pulses, as a principal gauge for evaluating each patient. However, it must be kept in mind that because he had no reliable timekeeping device the *swnw* could form only a rough estimate of pulse rate or of the force of the pulsations. The final "diagnosis" in each case was not given a name; instead, it was indicated simply by repeating the major clinical findings.[35] Clearly, most of the *swnw*'s examination techniques were designed to elucidate the state of the *metu*, and, by extension, the *wḫdw*. Even "surgical" conditions could be interpreted in this light.

The skin was subject to a wide range of obvious afflictions, including itch, boils, carbuncles, acne, burns, contusions, and purulent bites, wherever the *wḫdw* managed to surface. The Egyptians also thought that it caused baldness and white hair, and that both should be remedied.

Infections, such as smallpox, anthrax, and leprosy, which have been tentatively (but arguably) diagnosed in a few mummies, would also have been interpreted as the result of *wḫdw* that had risen to the body surface.

The number of remedies for them given in the Ebers and Hearst papyri hint that muscle spasms and limited joint mobility may have been common. Rheumatoid joint disease and the related disease of the spine, ankylosing spondylitis, are infrequent among mummies, but degenerative osteoarthritis and osteoporosis have been detected in older individuals. The pain and limited motion that are the principal symptoms of most musculoskeletal problems were viewed as caused by the effects of *wḫdw* in the *metu* that served the limbs, even in the absence of abnormal secretions or other evidence on the body's surface.

Disease carried to the head by its several *metu* included colds, deafness, earache, glossitis (inflammation of the tongue), pyorrhea (inflammation of the gums), loose teeth, and caries. The eye was subject to common disorders such as sties and other inflammations, and possibly strabismus (often called "squint" today), while the *swnw* also attempted to treat the pockets of fatty tissue (xanthelasma) that accumulate in the corner of the eye in people with certain patterns of fat metabolism. Trachoma, a form of blindness caused by infection of the conjunctiva by the micro-organism called *Chlamydia trachomatis*, seems to have been common on the banks of the Nile even five millennia ago, and night blindness is mentioned in the Ebers Papyrus. Some blindness was specifically attributed to the patient's sins, and required magic for its treatment. (Although harpists were usually—but not always—portrayed as blind, not much medical significance can be attached to such representations. Blind harpists may have been symbolic, or they may only illustrate an occupation that was suitable for the blind, since the Egyptians had no written musical notation that we know of.) Cataracts were so named because the eye was thought to become clouded by excessive water running out of the *metu* to the eye and down between the iris and the lens (the English use of "cataract" has a slightly different origin). Consequently, tears were thought to be beneficial because they released water, so that it could not accumulate in the *metu* of the eye and cause cataracts. Much of the *swnw*'s concern for the eyes may also have arisen from the eyes' association with the myth of the popular god Horus, which will be noted later in another medical context.[36]

Nervous system disorders are scarcely mentioned in the papyri. The Egyptians did not recognize the brain's contribution to the body's functioning, and no *metu* traveled to or from it. Although the author of the Smith Papyrus did note the relationship between certain cranial injuries and paralysis on the opposite side of the body, and between a broken neck and involuntary erection, he was an unusually thorough observer. Moreover, he could not have connected his observations specifically with the brain, since it was regarded as physiologically irrelevant. At least one ancient medical author may have observed a case of epilepsy (although other diagnoses are possible), even if he could not yet associate it with the central nervous system.

Pulse

Perhaps because the Egyptians regarded the heart as the body's principal organ, absolutely essential to life, and the major distributing center for *wḫdw*, they failed to recognize its role as a potential seat of disease; Western medicine, too, generally overlooked the heart as a possible disease site until the Greco-Roman humoral theory finally became moribund in the nineteenth century.[37] Although the *swnw* could palpate the pulse at several sites, he could not know that the blood circulates, nor could he differentiate blood vessels from nerves and tendons. He only seems to have recognized that the pulse is an important diagnostic sign, linked to cardiac activity and, especially, to the condition of the *metu*.

The author of the Ebers Papyrus noted that the pulse could be expected to disappear when his patient fainted. Ancient physicians also seem to have been able to detect several possible abnormalities of the heartbeat: extra beats (extrasystoles), identifiable by what they called "forgotten beats;" left ventricular enlargement (hypertrophy), now recognizable in retrospect because the *swnw* reported that the heart impulse on the chest wall was displaced to the left of its usual position; and the weak thready pulse that would later be associated with heart failure. "Flooding of the heart," which the *swnw* attributed to excessive salivation,[38] may have been only a metaphor (I hesitate to exploit the word "imaginary"), but it might also have represented some cardiac disease that today would be interpreted as heart failure.

Although mummies have shown clear evidence of arteriosclerosis, this condition would have been beyond the *swnw*'s comprehension. He sometimes did see an association among disorders of the liver, lungs, and heart, but he could not have understood the patient's symptoms as the result of blood or fluid congestion in those organs and elsewhere, especially since he was unaware that the blood circulates within a closed system. The Ebers Papyrus reports a case in which "something entering the patient's mouth" produced pains in his arm, breast, and heart, so that "death threatened him." It is too tempting to diagnose this retrospectively as a case of angina pectoris, although it is certainly possible; the ancient author surmised only that when the offending cause had descended to the lower intestine would the patient be cured,[39] a prediction that probably stems from the postulate that the *wḫdw* could be flushed out with the feces.

Because air was regarded as essential for the life of both gods and men, the lungs were considered sufficiently important to the body's needs in the next life to warrant separate preservation in canopic jars or with the mummy. However, most were not preserved well enough for microscopic study today (save for the few that have shown unmistakable evidence of tuberculosis and pneumoconioses).[40]

Liver disease was seldom recognized separately, presumably because it could not be, although the Ebers Papyrus notes that a liver (or spleen) that is too full of blood can produce all diseases; after all, it was served by many *metu*. Since the organ was routinely preserved separately, it might have been observed more closely than many others. Still, only two or three cases of possibly symptomatic gallstones have been found, while one autopsied liver has revealed cirrhosis secondary to schistosomiasis.

The central role of the gastrointestinal tract among the *swnw*'s physiological concepts led to its recognition as a major site of illness, but the association was probably more often assumed than real, considering the gut's hypothetical central role as the source of *wḫdw*. Although the stomach and intestines were also regularly preserved, the rapid onset of their post-mortem decay has precluded finding more than a mere scattering of barely recognizable disease in them. The intestinal complaints most often mentioned in the medical papyri are anal itching, bloating, hemorrhoids, and rectal prolapse. Generalized abdominal discomfort was related to incomplete digestion, especially after overeating. Similar dyspeptic symptoms were also attributed to the presence of the ever-dangerous "Blood-eater" in the stomach. Finally, constipation, or at least fear of it, may have been widespread, if the number of remedies for it in the medical papyri is a valid gauge of its prevalence or of concern about it.[41]

Probably because the kidneys were out of the embalmer's field of view or easy reach, they are not mentioned in the medical papyri. The *swnw*'s urological knowledge was limited largely to functional disorders, such as urinary retention, bed-wetting, cystitis (if that is the diagnosis most clearly suggested by complaints of lower abdominal pain accompanied by painful urination), priapism (persistent erection), and incontinence of urine following severe neck trauma and quadriplegia. The papyri do not mention urinary tract stones, although a few have been found in mummies. Gonorrhea may have been present in pharaonic Egypt, but probably not syphilis.[42] Because urine is the most voluminous secretion of the body, symptoms related to it and its associated organs could easily be interpreted in terms of disordered *metu*.

The Egyptians must have expected the *swnw* and other healers to postpone their deaths when possible, but they were not particularly morbid or fatalistic about the end of life. Indeed, the thought and energy they directed toward their hopes and rituals for the deceased and his life in the next world suggest the opposite, as does "The Dispute between a Man and his *Ba*." As John Wilson has noted, in pharaonic Egypt death "promised every good man a happy eternity. . . . Self-assurance, optimism, and a lust for life produced an energetic assertion of eternally continuing life rather than elaborate defenses against death."[43] But Egyptians were well aware that death constantly threatened them, if only because they lived rather precariously on the edge of an uncompromising desert where they were totally dependent on the Nile's sporadically unreliable annual flooding. Even if they regarded their life spans as determined by fate or the gods, they could still deny death psychologically, as we do, and try to fend it off a little longer with a *swnw*'s help.

Few, if any, modern pathophysiological concepts can be recognized among the Egyptian medical texts, just as only a few modern diagnoses can be recognized in preserved ancient bodies and organs. Save for, perhaps, several parasitic diseases, however, we cannot doubt that many diseases familiar to modern Americans were present as early as the Old Kingdom, although their incidences undoubtedly differed from those we see today. The *swnw* could follow only his own rather speculative concepts of how the body works, and of how it responds to disease and to treatment, as he worked to postpone the inevitable.

5

THE *SWNW'S* MEDICINES

All three categories of ancient Egyptian healers—magicians, priests, and lay *swnw*—shared many of the same therapeutic methods. (We do not know how their patients chose among the three groups, or even if they had any choice in the matter at all.) Both the magico-religious and the empirico-rational traditions relied on spells, amulets, healing statues, sanctifed water, and dream revelation, albeit to different degrees. The priests and magicians also used many of the *swnw*'s diagnostic methods, and they undoubtedly shared his pathophysiological concepts of the *metu* and *wḫdw*.

The various practitioners differed most in that a hallmark of the lay *swnw* was his therapeutic reliance chiefly on drugs and minor surgery. He did exploit the supernatural from time to time, but most of his methods for balancing the contents of the *metu* were based on the therapeutic logic outlined in the last chapter, even if some of his remedies had additional magical connotations.

The notion of health as something positive may have originated in an underlying uneasiness shared by all Egyptians. They lived in a land in which the life-giving Nile could be unpredictably derelict, a land subject to the whims of gods and tax collectors, a land where internal disorder and occasional foreign invaders might leave long-lasting scars on the people's health and general well-being. In such circumstances, magic would have provided important prophylactic measures in addition to its presumed curative properties. The maintenance of stability as a preventive strategy was a legitimate goal of kings, bureaucrats, priests—and the *swnw*. For instance, both the physician and the pharaoh recognized the stabilizing value of adequate dietary intake for maintaining normality. The *swnw* depended on it explicitly for enhancing the healing process, as in the surgeon's recommendation to leave certain patients "at their mooring stakes," a metaphor for stabilizing the body while it healed. Similarly, the king had to make sure that his subjects were well fed in order to assure political stability and optimum productivity.

Magico-religious prevention and common sense, as well as professional medical care, were of as much concern to the average Egyptian as to his political and religious leaders, and to his village *swnw*. A number of aphorisms, even if they were written down as late as Ptolemaic and Roman times, reflect all these approaches to illness and its treatment. For instance, the importance of religion is evident in: "A timely remedy is to prevent illness by having the greatness of the god in your heart." The common-sense approach underlies injunctions such as: "Do not pamper yourself when you are young, lest you be weak when you are old," "Do not be despondent when you are ill; your [death] is not made yet," and, "There is no tooth that rots yet stays in place." Finally, there are aphorisms that focus on the appropriate use of medicines. Some encourage compliance with the *swnw*'s directions: "Do not slight a small illness for which there is a remedy; use the remedy," "Do not scorn a remedy that you can use," and "Do not say 'My illness has passed, I will not use medication.' " Indeed, the role of the *swnw* was seen as indispensable: "A remedy is effective only through the hand of its physician." However one chose to approach it, "All sickness is troublesome; the wise man knows how to be sick."[1]

In the long run, of course, maintaining the body's *status quo*, with or without the aid of magic, would never be enough all by itself. The healing professions can be visualized as having grown out of a perception that the successful cure of illness required active intervention. As we have seen, several ancient wound treatments were practical solutions to clearly evident problems. But, as we have also seen, the *swnw* lacked the kind of information about internal disorders and their causes that we possess today. Instead, he had to rely on a physiological theory to which he readily adapted a wide range of drugs from the plant, mineral, and animal kingdoms.

A great many ancient remedies have survived in the Egyptian medical papyri. They are probably the oldest compendia of prescriptions ever written; some passages in them were almost certainly first composed during the Old Kingdom. Just afterward, during the First Intermediate Period, the earliest datable prescriptions yet found anywhere were inscribed (about 2100 B.C.) in Sumerian cuneiform on a clay tablet found in Iraq, at Nippur, about 100 miles south of Baghdad. It lists ingredients for eight poultices and seven internal remedies. Some of the raw materials were also used in Egyptian medicines, but the Sumerian tablet does not specify the symptoms for which each prescription is appropriate, nor does it specify the amounts of each ingredient to be used, although the Sumerians already possessed well-developed numerical and measuring systems by then. The tablet, which contains no magical spells, seems to represent drugs developed in an empirico-rational tradition like that expressed in the Ebers Papyrus.[2] Several Near Eastern civilizations in Mesopotamia and Anatolia probably had some influence on Egyptian therapeutics, but no definite links between them have yet been reported.[3]

Although most ancient Egyptian remedies can now be recognized as incapable of providing definitive cures, or even selectively palliative therapy, it would be unfair to represent them either as placebos or as pioneering clinical trials in the modern sense. Egyptian drug therapy should probably be regarded as having developed gradually from magical roots into an empirical and rational system that was self-perpetuating to the extent that the body was able to heal itself. That is, the *swnw* had no reason to believe that his drugs were not beneficial to his patients who recovered after taking them. It was the underlying physiological premises of pharaonic pharmacology that were faulty, not the ancient physician's applications of them.

The *swnw* seems to have differentiated, to some extent at least, between remedies he thought affected the *metu* and those with more explicitly magical rationales, such as the mouse. Skinned whole mice have been found in the stomachs of children buried in a predynastic cemetery, perhaps administered as a treatment of last resort. Mouse fat is recommended in the Ebers Papyrus "to relax stiffness" and a mouse head to remedy earaches. A rotten mouse is the chief ingredient of a Hearst Papyrus ointment that would keep the hair from turning white. During the reign of Nero (54–68 A.D.), the Greek physician Dioscorides noted that whole mice would dry children's saliva, and that chopped mice were useful for scorpion bites. Two thousand years later, in 1924, skinned whole mice were being used for the treatment of both urinary incontinence and whooping cough in rural England.[4] From the Old Kingdom to twentieth-century Britain, the healers who used them thought that these murine treatments were sound, an assessment that is probably valid in view of what those healers knew and observed. Besides, the *swnw*, like many of his successors ever since, often treated symptoms that were inherently evanescent, not their underlying causes; any treatment for such symptoms is bound to be judged effective.

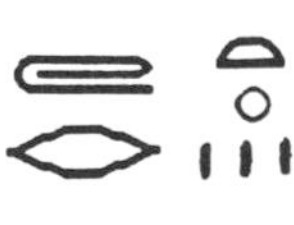

Prescription, or remedy

The drug prescriptions given in the medical papyri have essentially the same structural organization as is used today: the "inscription" (the name and amount of the drug's ingredients); the "subscription" (directions for preparing the medicine for administration to the patient); and the "signature" (instructions to the patient for taking his medicine). Although today's subscriptions are instructions to pharmacists, their profession was unknown in ancient Egypt, where physicians (or their servants) prepared most remedies,[5] probably using their own mortars and pestles[6] to grind them.

Because the stylized eye of the falcon-headed god Horus represented unity and, therefore, wholeness and health, the *swnw* used it to symbolize his intention to restore his patient. According to an ancient myth, the god's eye was torn apart in a fight with his uncle, the wicked god Seth, but it was put back together by the ibis-headed god Thoth to become the *uadjat*, "the whole eye." Consequently, the parts of the *uadjat* (variously transliterated as *wedjat* or *oudjat*, and pronounced accordingly) came to be used as a practical shorthand to represent parts of the whole when listing amounts of each ingredient to be used in preparing specific drug mixtures (see Figure 16). Each part of the eye symbol represents some fraction of 64 parts, and was, therefore, convenient for indicating proportional parts of the whole.[7] The fractions shown in Figure 16 add up to only 63/64, so it has been presumed that Thoth magically supplied the remainder (but there is little real need to account for all 64 sixty-fourths). The *uadjet* was also used to express fractions of the *ḥeḳat*-measure for grains; one-*ḥeḳat* vessels have been found to contain about four quarts (actually, 4.54 liters). Measures of less than 1/64 of a *ḥeḳat* were expressed in terms of the *ro*, 1/320 of a *ḥeḳat*, or about 15 milliliters, half an ounce. Liquids like beer and honey, as well as grains, were

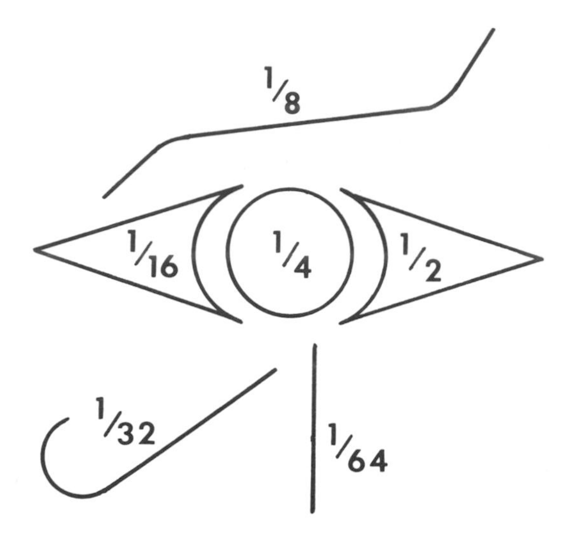

FIGURE 16. The symbols used for volume measures, as derived from the eye of the falcon-headed god Horus.

commonly measured by the *hin*, about 1/10 of a *ḥeḳat*, although actual measurements show that it was closer to one pint (0.503 liter).

Pan scales had been used for many purposes since at least the Old Kingdom, including weighing drugs,[8] although medicines were also made up by proportional volumes. The drug amounts specified in the medical papyri with *uadjet* notations were probably meant simply as proportional parts of the final whole.[9] That accurate measurements of drug ingredients and of dose were considered relevant and important has been inferred from the fact that about 60 percent of the approximately 1350 prescriptions in all the medical papyri specify the amounts of each ingredient. Drugs for oral administration were most often prescribed in terms of the half-ounce *ro*, which was the size of a modern tablespoonful—a mouthful. Thus, medical arithmetic probably began as a tool for preparing and dispensing drugs in convenient dose sizes. The Egyptians' mathematical methods were cumbersome and inefficient, but they were sufficient for this and many other computational purposes.[10]

Our principal sources of information about the *swnw*'s drugs are the Ebers and Hearst papyri. Unlike the Smith Papyrus, which seems to be the work of one author or two at most (as well as of an annotator), these documents are collations from various sources. Both manuscripts date from the early New Kingdom (about 1550 B.C.), but reflect at least some practices already current in the Old Kingdom. The Ebers Papyrus is, according to its translator, Bendix Ebbell, a compilation (including two parts called *The Physician's Secret* and *The Collection on Expelling the Wḫdw*) based on "a definite and closely considered plan, care being taken to include the most different diseases that a 'physician' should treat."[11] The Hearst Papyrus is organized along different lines; its compiler, who may have prepared it as a reference for everyday use by a village *swnw*, seems to have been more interested in the drugs he listed than in the organ system approach to disease and its treatment employed by the compiler of the Ebers Papyrus, although some of the Hearst author's text is arranged by categories of illness.[12]

The two other major—although much shorter—medical documents from ancient Egypt are the Kahun Gynecological Papyrus[13] and the Chester Beatty VI Papyrus, which deals chiefly with disorders of the lower intestinal tract.[14] (The Berlin Papyrus No. 3038 of about 1350 B.C., which is not otherwise discussed here because it is available only in German, appears to add little if anything that is substantive to the range of remedies described in the Ebers and Hearst documents.) A few medical (i.e., nonmagical) prescriptions are known from other sources, but excepting two for cough and earache, they do not mention the symptoms for which the remedies are indicated.[15]

Because the Hearst Papyrus lists the amounts of each ingredient required for oral drug preparations more often than the amounts to be included in topically applied medications, the modern pharmacologist-historian Chauncey Leake inferred that the *swnw* used more care in preparing oral medications because they could be expected to have more systemic effects, than in making remedies for topical application (including enemas and rectal or vaginal suppositories). The Smith Papyrus does show that the *swnw* thought that the *metu* were capable of "taking up" (i.e., absorbing) ingested remedies as well as "the rotten stuff" that produced disease. Leake also reasoned that the *swnw* perceived that the intensity of drug effect was proportional to drug dose, and that they took care to avoid preparing mixtures that might result in clinically significant overdoses. Finally, Leake concluded that the *swnw* also knew that some drugs were more potent than others that produced the same effect.[16] (However, Leake's inferences must be regarded as tentative; I can neither verify nor reject them on the basis of the information and texts that are available.)

Only 28 percent of the 260 prescriptions given in the Hearst Papyrus contain one or more supposedly active ingredients that have been identified satisfactorily; they represent about 65 percent of all the active ingredients given in the document. By contrast, about 95 percent of Ebers Papyrus prescriptions contain one or more identifiable raw materials (whether "active" or not), but most also contain at least one untranslatable ingredient. However, virtually all prescriptions in both compendia contain explicit instructions for their method of administration (see Table 2); almost three-fourths were designed for topical application, and one-fourth for oral administration. Most of the latter were meant to be taken once a day for four days.

About half of all the drug ingredients listed in the Appendix were used in one or more external wound treatments. Ointments alone were recommended for 42 percent of the 45 different injuries described in the Smith Surgical Papyrus, and were used in conjunction with operative or manipulative techniques in another 44 percent; most of these medicines contained honey. Of the 29 different materials recommended for therapeutic or diagnostic use in the Kahun Gynecological Papyrus, 14 percent were to be administered into the vagina by fumigation in smoke, and 31 percent by manual application; 24 percent were to be given by mouth; and another 24 percent were for external application on the body's surface. Several gargles and solid substances that may have been meant to be chewed without swallowing, usually to freshen the breath, are found in the Ebers and other papyri. Thus, the *swnw* could choose a route of

TABLE 2. Routes of administration, when specified, in 815 nonmagical prescriptions given in the Ebers Papyrus and 260 prescriptions in the Hearst Papyrus.

	In Ebers Papyrus	***In Hearst Papyrus***
For Oral Administration	28.83%	26.63%
To be Applied Topically:		
For Local Effects on Skin, Rectum, Vagina, Etc.	*(63.31%)*	
For Effects Elsewhere in the Body	(7.61%)	
Total	70.92%	73.13%
To be Inhaled	0.12%	0.12%
To be Introduced in Smoke to the Vagina	0.12%	0.12%

drug administration that was best adapted to his patient's particular problem, more or less regardless of the specific therapeutic properties ascribed to the drug. That is, the *swnw* seem to have distinguished among the ways in which medicines were prepared in order to expedite their entry into disordered *metu* vessels: as pills, liquids, suppositories, or topical ointments, any route that would facilitate selective attacks on diseases residing in particular target *metu*.

Some of the raw materials specified in the medical papyri were used as vehicles in which the "active ingredients" were dissolved or suspended, or which permitted them to be compressed into solid lozenges or pills. The range of vehicles used in Egyptian medicines (see Table 3) would have dissolved materials that are soluble in water or alcohol, or both. Honey, after water the most common drug ingredient, must have been thought to be therapeutically active in many prescriptions, as it was in the wound ointments described in the Smith Papyrus; the Ebers Papyrus provides no clues to any presumed pharmacological properties of this extremely important component of the ancient Egyptians' materia medica.

Table 4 lists the 25 presumably "active" raw ingredients mentioned most frequently in the Ebers Papyrus, again including honey because of its ambiguous position as vehicle or active medicine. It would not be profitable to attempt to correlate these ingredients with modern pharmacological concepts of their therapeutic value, if only because the drugs' precise clinical applications by the *swnw* are not sufficiently well understood, not to mention the philological difficulties involved in trans-

TABLE 3. Materials used primarily as solvents or diluents in medicines described in the Ebers Papyrus. (For details of each, see the Appendix.)

WATER or DEW		53.5 %
HONEY (but ? "active")		30.3 %
BEER		14.5 %
WHITE OIL		14.5 %
FAT or GREASE:		
Bovine	[3.8 %]	
Goose	[5.0 %]	14.3 %
Other	[5.5 %]	
WINE		5.2 %
MILK or CREAM		4.6 %
BEESWAX		4.4 %

lating the Egyptian words. On the other hand, we will shortly examine some of the general clinical indications for which the *swnw* prescribed several drugs. The Appendix identifies and cross-indexes as many of the ingredients given in the papyri as possible, along with their apparent therapeutic applications.

Table 4 also points up the apparently conflicting uses of some drug materials as both laxatives *and* antidiarrheals. Of all the materials listed in the table, colocynth is the only strong laxative that was not also used in remedies for diarrhea. If honey had been used chiefly as a vehicle for binding medications, it would not be surprising to see both kinds of clinical actions ascribed to drugs containing it, but other ingredients that were also used for both antithetical purposes, such as yellow ochre and juniper, were never used as vehicles, so the Egyptians' understanding of honey's therapeutic properties remains moot.

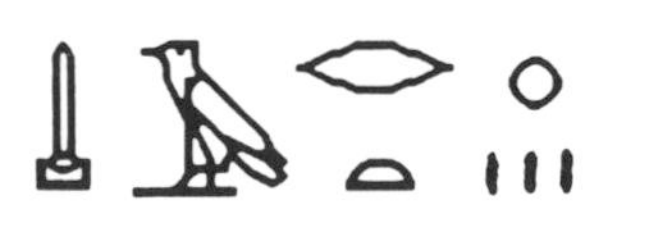

Djaret

Most perplexing of all is the plant drug called *djaret* (probably pronounced more or less as it looks), which has never been adequately and convincingly identified, although it appears in more recipes than any ingredient except water and honey. If, as has been suggested, it was the true opium poppy, *Papaver somniferum* (although it was not found in Egypt before the New Kingdom), it might have counteracted diarrhea, but it would not have promoted bowel movements. On the other hand, *djaret* has also been tentatively identified as colocynth, but that would certainly not have ameliorated diarrhea. A third suggested translation, carob, has little if any effect as either an antidiarrheal or a laxative. (The Egyptians usually employed other words for colocynth and carob, and they may have had another, *špnn*, (pronounced *shepenn*), for opium.)[17] The *swnw* may well have used *djaret* for both kinds of effects on the bowels if he was less concerned with its actual than with its presumed effects, as was probably the case.

Perhaps as many as a third of all the drug ingredients listed in the Appendix have clearly identifiable pharmacological properties. About half of them do stimulate the bowels, and a few are weak emetics, antidiarrheals, and astringents (agents that make tissues contract, arrest secretions, or stop bleeding, as styptics do). Several were regarded as

TABLE 4. Drug ingredients given most often in the Ebers Papyrus, and their use in laxatives(*) and/or in antidiarrheal agents(**). (For details of each, see the Appendix.)

Ingredient	%	Laxative	Antidiarrheal	Combined
HONEY (? as solvent)	30.3 %	*	**	
djaret	14.6 %	*	**	
FRANKINCENSE	14.1 %	*		
SALT, NORTHERN	9.3 %	*		[10.4 %]*
SALT	1.1 %	*		
DATES	6.9 %	*		[9.6 %]*
DATE WINE	2.7 %	*		
STIBIUM or GALENA (ores of antimony, lead)	8.2 %			
YELLOW OCHRE (iron oxides)	8.2 %	*	**	
CUMIN and/or AMMI seeds	7.7 %	*		
JUNIPER	6.2 %	*	**	
NATRON	4.6%			[6.2 %]
RED NATRON	1.5 %			
ACACIA juice, leaves	6.1 %			
COLOCYNTH	5.3 %	*		
FIGS	5.2 %	*		
SYCOMORE FIGS	5.2 %	*	**	
MYRRH	5.2 %			
RED OCHRE (iron oxides)	4.9 %			
MALACHITE (a copper salt)	4.6 %	*		
PIGNONS (pine seeds)	4.6 %	*	**	
SEBESTEN fruit	4.5 %	*		
BALANITES OIL	4.2 %			
RUSH-NUTS	4.2 %	*		
CALOTROPIS (? CELERY)	3.6 %			

carminatives (agents that expel gas from the intestinal tract, a now obsolete drug class further described in the Appendix) into our own century. At least one plant drug, hyoscyamus, which still grows on the banks of the Nile, might have caused sedation and perhaps a modest degree of analgesia. But unless we can determine that drugs with known pharmacological effects (other than catharsis) were given to patients with given symptoms considerably more often than drugs with no known selectivity, we cannot conclude that the *swnw* were prescribing them for reasons associated with the drugs' special properties.

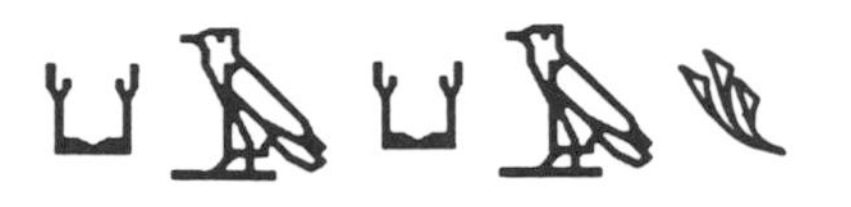

Castor bean plant

Only for ricinus, the castor bean, did the compiler of the Ebers Papyrus (or any other, for that matter) include what he took to be a complete description of its therapeutic benefits:

> *To know what is made with the ricinus-plant according to that which was found in old writings as something useful to men: if its roots are crushed in water and applied to a head which is ill, then he will get well immediately like one who is not ill. But if a little of its seed is chewed with beer by a man with looseness in his excrements [i.e., diarrhea], then it expels the disease in the belly of the man. Further the hair of a woman is made to grow by means of its seed: it is ground, mixed together and put into oil by the woman, who shall rub her head therewith. Further its oil in its seed is used to annoint one who [suffers] from the rose [?] with bad putrid [??], then [??] the skin as [in] one whom nothing has befallen. But he is treated by rubbing the aforesaid for 10 days, rubbing in very early in the morning, until it is expelled. Really excellent, [proved] many times!*[18]

It is not possible to comment usefully on castor oil's purported effect on the scalp. The use of a dependable cathartic in the treatment of diarrhea might seem irrational at first, but if the goal of therapy with the drug was to hasten expulsion of the *wḫdw* that was causing the diarrhea in the first place, and not simply the cessation of diarrhea, then a dose of castor beans would seem entirely reasonable to the *swnw*. If that is true, then it might have seemed equally rational to prescribe yellow ochre or juniper for both diarrhea and constipation.

None of the remedies identifiable in the medical papyri is especially dangerous in a single dose unless taken in large amounts (e.g., lead and antimony), and there is no good evidence that the Egyptians used explicit poisons for legal or illegal homicide. No definite traces of poisons have been detected in medical texts, on arrow points, or in mummies. Apparent human sacrifices, possibly killed by poison, were buried with the earliest Egyptian and Nubian rulers, but the practice seems to have stopped by the end of Dynasty I. A single unconfirmed clue in a papyrus in the Louvre (the admonition "Do not pronounce the name of [a certain god], under pain of [punishment by] the peach") has suggested that peach pits may have been used to execute persons guilty of having betrayed liturgical secrets; presumably they would have died of cyanide poisoning, as is expected from overdoses of apricot pit extracts or apple seeds today. However, most scholars agree that poison was not used for execution, and that the most frequent poisonings were accidental, caused by snakes or scorpions, or perhaps by atropine-like plants such as *Hyoscyamus* or *Datura* species, although those plants cannot be guaranteed to cause death even if they do make the patient quite sick for some time.[19]

Animal parts and products appear in 42 percent of all prescriptions in the Ebers Papyrus (see Table 5). About one-third of those mentioned are of fat (in 4.5 percent of all prescriptions) and grease (9.5 percent), both of which were probably used as vehicles. About 27 percent of the materials derived from animals were body products and excretions: urine (in 0.4 percent of all recipes), eggs (1.5 percent), milk (4.3 percent), dung (5.2 percent), and the milk of a woman who had borne a male child

TABLE 5. Animal parts and products used to make drugs described in the Ebers Papyrus. (For details of each, see the Appendix.)

BLOOD	HEART
BRAINS	LIVER; GALL
HEAD, EAR, EYES, TEETH, HORNS, SKULL	SPLEEN
	TESTES and UTERUS
BONE and MARROW	EGGS
SKIN and HAIR	URINE or DUNG
MEAT	MILK, of OX or ASS
FAT and GREASE	MILK, of MOTHER OF A MALE CHILD

(1.7 percent). Structural components of animal bodies, such as blood, bones, and meat, were used in compounding 16 percent of the Ebers prescriptions.

Fats and greases might have provided suitable emollient bases for ointments, but none of the other animal products listed in the table has any selective therapeutic value, with the possible exception of liver when prescribed for night blindness.[20] The amount of Vitamin A in liver would have been sufficient to correct the responsible deficiency if the patient continued to take the remedy for a while at least. But in general one must conclude that the value of the animal parts used in making Egyptian remedies (other than fat-based ointments) was more magical than physiological, and that it resembled folk healing practices that have survived into our own time. In addition, Sigerist has raised the possibility that seemingly bizzare remedies, such as ass's head and pig's tooth, should not be taken as literal equivalents of those objects, that they may have been only slang or jargon terms for entirely different materials.[21]

The range of animal species from which those parts were taken is shown in Table 6. It, too, supports the conclusion that animal ingredients (other than beef fat) were included because of their magical or religious associations, not because they possessed any selectivity of pharmacological action, such as that of malachite and honey.

Other ancient Egyptian drugs were used quite rationally, but not from any modern pharmacological premise, nor from any that were corollaries of the concept of the *metu*. Because any special qualities inherent in a given organism were thought to reside in its tissues, stallion saliva

TABLE 6. Animal species used in medicines given in the Ebers Papyrus. (For details of each, see the Appendix.)

Major		*Infrequent*	
COW	Mouse	Ostrich	Frog
GOOSE	Goat	Pigeon	Lizards
ASS	Sheep	Pelican	Snakes
MAN	Bat	Raven	Tortoise
CAT	Hippopotamus		Crocodile
PIG	Antelope species		
	Dog		
	Several species of Fish and Insects		

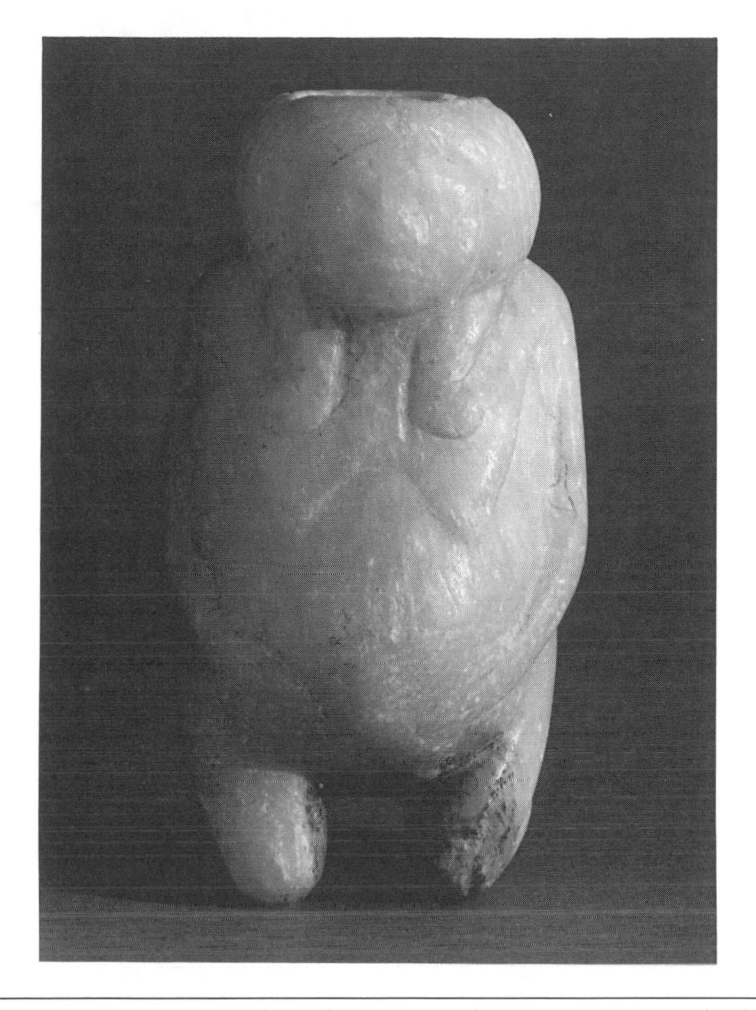

FIGURE 17. Alabaster bottle in the form of a kneeling woman, made about 1570-1293 B.C., and probably used as a container for a skin lotion to be used during pregnancy. (Courtesy, Museum of Fire Arts, Boston, 02.525, gift of the estate of Mrs. S. D. Warren)

was administered to stimulate a woman's libido when her husband thought it necessary; the skin of an agile antelope was applied to a stiff foot; and the urine of a pregnant woman was sprinkled on grain fields to stimulate crop growth (just as grain was used in the pregnancy tests described in Chapter Three). Similarly, secretions and organs, such as semen and placenta, were thought to possess the fertilizing properties of their sources, just as fish heads were assumed to drain off headaches and hogs' eyes to cure blindness. And, because the goddess Isis had nursed her son Horus back to life by treating his burns with her milk, so the milk of a woman who had had a male child was highly regarded because it could both transmit the special powers implied by the myth and guarantee a strong constitution to the person who drank it; it might even induce the birth of a male child to women who drank it.

Finally, disagreeable substances like dung and urine were expected to repel evil spirits who had made a patient ill, just as aromatic substances might attract benevolent spirits who would cast out the evil spirits responsible for a patient's disease. All of this was, of course, the kind of analogous magic that Frazer calls sympathetic, although the *swnw* who used such implicit rationales were not using magic in quite the same way that the healing priests and magicians used spells and incantations. In the end, of course, the healing magic of ancient Egypt was probably like that of ancient Greece, magic which G.E.R. Lloyd has described as assessed not by its results but by its appropriateness.[22]

The philological difficulties encountered in translating texts like the Ebers and Hearst papyri compound the difficulties in analyzing the pharmacological effects and the clinical value of the *swnw*'s medicines today. That task is further complicated by the necessity of understanding his drugs in *his* terms, and of forgetting our own criteria for assessing therapeutic efficacy. Past historical judgements on ancient Egyptian drugs have ranged from worthless[23] to the conclusion that the *swnw* prescribed according to "predetermined modes of action, rather than as an individual healer of his patients, a concept that emerged in the Hippocratic school [in the fifth century B.C.]."[24] But it should not be forgotten that many medicines first used on the banks of the Nile were still in use there and elsewhere in modern times, which suggests that they were judged to be successful as remedies over many generations and in many cultures.

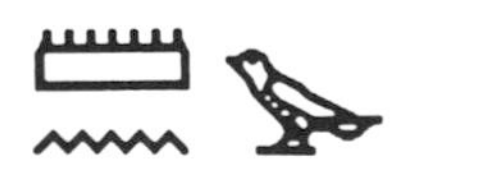

To be sick

The clinical indications for the 842 nonmagical prescriptions given in the Ebers Papyrus are summarized by the organ systems associated with each in Table 7.

TABLE 7. Clinical classification of drug usages given in the Ebers Papyrus.

Drugs for Disorders of:	***Percent of All Recipes***
RESPIRATORY TRACT AND HEART	4.6 %
HEAD, EARS, NOSE, AND MOUTH	6.2 %
FEMALE ORGANS	6.2 %
GENITOURINARY TRACT	6.8 %
SUPERFICIAL SKIN WOUNDS	9.5 %
EYES	11.2 %
LIMBS, JOINTS, AND SPINE	13.7 %
SKIN AND HAIR	15.7 %
GASTROINTESTINAL TRACT	26.2 %
With excess *wḫdw*	[11.5 %]
With obstructed bowels	[14.7 %]

The Ebers and Hearst papyri share about one-third of their prescriptions, and neither is all-inclusive. Both documents are interpretable within the same general framework of physiological and therapeutic knowledge, even if they differ in some respects (for instance, no eye remedies are found among the Hearst prescriptions). Thus, although the Hearst Papyrus cannot be analyzed in parallel with the Ebers Papyrus, both reflect the same principles of medical practice.

Compared to the Ebers Papyrus, the Hearst Papyrus contains many more prescriptions that are explicitly intended to remove or expel *wḫdw* from the body as a whole or from specific parts of it. For instance, one remedy is for expelling "sickness from all members," eight (3.1 percent of all 260) are aimed at stimulating urination, and nine (3.5 percent) are, similarly, for expelling fluids from the body. In addition, 42 (16.1 percent) are said to cool, relieve, soothe, or freshen the *metu*. If the Hearst Papyrus was indeed intended to be a practical *vade mecum* for everyday use, such instructions would have provided practical guidelines for the *swnw*; the same concepts are clearly meant in the Ebers Papyrus prescriptions but are not stated there so explicitly.

It is tempting to translate, or interpret, some of the terms used in the medical papyri as having specific modern analogues. For instance, one might wish to interpret the Hearst author's "seizures" and "jumping in the limbs" as our "epilepsy," but that could be hazardous, because the *swnw*-scribe might actually have observed convulsions in febrile patients, or he might have meant some effect of *wḫdw* in the affected limbs, one that he could not observe directly but only conjectured in some way consistent with the theory of the *metu*. It would be equally presumptuous to interpret "swellings of limbs" as joint disease, or prescriptions "causing one to urinate" as remedies for prostatic enlargement or for the edema commonly associated with heart failure.[25] It is certain that the *swnw* could not make direct observations of the lungs or body cavities in his patients. He probably made his inferences about the heart solely on the evidence of the pulse, if he used any direct evidence at all (after all, the concept of the *metu* required that the heart be the major distribution center for the pathogenic *wḫdw*).

Although just over 70 percent of Egyptian remedies were designed for topical administration, more than a tenth of these were thought to exert their effects elsewhere in the body, such as drugs applied to the anus for women with diseases of the uterus, or to the skin for expelling *wḫdw* from the *metu*. In general, the greatest proportion of oral preparations was prescribed for intestinal disorders, including disturbances of the *metu* and excessive *wḫdw*. Perhaps the *swnw* really thought that he was applying his oral medications topically to the interior of the gastrointestinal tract, where much of his physiological thinking was focussed; even if he did think that drugs could be absorbed from the intestinal tract into the *metu* ducts, it is not certain that he could also recognize that they might be redistributed to other parts of the body. A corollary hypothesis is Sigerist's interpretation of Egyptian drugs as "internal amulets" that were thought to exert their powers—medicinal *and* magical—from inside the body.[26]

Unfortunately, we cannot assess the extent to which the *swnw* actually relied on any given remedy among the many available to him for the treatment of any given condition among all his patients. The Ebers prescriptions contain an average of 4.2 ingredients in each, including vehicles, ranging from one to 37 (in a clearly magical mixture for curing impotence). Consequently, we can base our conclusions about the ancient physicians' reliance on any given drug ingredients for any specific conditions only on the frequencies with which they appear among the prescriptions for such conditions. This approach assumes that the more often a given substance appears in the prescriptions, the more satisfactory it was thought to have been for doing the job assigned to it, regardless of the criteria for assessing its efficacy. This assumption may not be completely valid, but it does provide a convenient working hypothesis.

Tables 8-A and 8-B list the raw ingredients that were included most often among the Ebers Papyrus prescriptions (in 10–20 percent, 20–40 percent, or more than 40 percent of each clinical category) for both clearly recognizable organ-related illnesses (Table 8-A) and for those explicitly described as disorders of the *wḫdw* in various anatomic areas or as divinely produced disease in the belly (Table 8-B). Materials like *djaret*, frankincense, dates, and salt that appear frequently among remedies for several unrelated disease categories can be regarded as having been aimed relatively nonselectively at diverse physiologically unrelated conditions. On the other hand, a very few raw ingredients were prescribed only (or primarily) for one kind of illness; for instance, stibium (although the correct translation may be galena; see both in the Appendix) was used almost exclusively for afflictions of the eye. However, it should also be recognized that, while *djaret* was used for a wide range of symptoms referable to many organ systems, as well as for unseen disorders of the *metu* or those caused by the gods, it was a favored ingredient for remedies designed to alleviate intestinal symptoms, even those that had purely magical causes. The major therapeutic uses and selectivities, if any can be detected, of identifiable ancient Egyptian drug ingredients are given in the Appendix.

A few potential plant remedies are puzzling because they do *not* appear in the major medical papyri, although they must have been familiar to the Egyptians since they used such plants in their decorative motifs. The most baffling omission is that of the mandrake (it was probably the North African species *Mandragora autumnalis* which grew in ancient Egypt, not the more familiar European one, *M. officinarum*). It must have been well known to the Egyptians who painted its distinctive fruits on their vases and jars.[27] The plant belongs to the botanical family Solanaceae, which produces several alkaloids that affect the nervous system. Like its botanical relatives the henbanes and the nightshades, the mandrake also contains substances resembling atropine, hyoscyamine, and scopolamine. It had a long-lived reputation as a sedative, analgesic, and aphrodisiac; the latter property was exploited by the earliest Hebrews long before their captivity in Egypt,[28] but there is no evidence that mandrake was used for any pharmacological purpose in Egypt. During the Renaissance the ancient plant began to disappear from European medical usage when its historic medical properties were found to be not very dependable.[29] Although it was not mentioned in any of the Egyptian medical papyri, it would be surprising if the *swnw* neglected the mandrake simply because it was not uniformly effective; indeed, most of his drugs undoubtedly did not live up to his expectations from time to time.

Although as many as a third of all Egyptian remedies could have had some effect on the gastrointestinal tract (as emetics, laxatives, antidi-

Ingredients included in 10–20% of Recipes for each CLINICAL INDICATION:	***In 20–40%***	***More than 40%***
POOR VISION: Balm of Mecca, Marrow, Myrrh, Sagapen	*djaret* Malachite	Stibium
EYE TRAUMA & TUMORS: Aloe, Balm of Mecca, Blood, *djaret*, Dung, Frankincense, Red Ochre, Yellow Ochre	Malachite	Stibium
EYE INFLAMMATIONS: Aloe, *djaret*, Ink-Powder, Malachite, Myrrh, Red Ochre, Stibium, Yellow Ochre		
HEAD PAINS: Camphor, Cumin, Coriander, *djaret*, Fish Bones, Juniper, Ladanum, Natron, Pine Products		Frankincense
SORE LIMBS: *djaret*, Figs, Natron, Myrrh, Pine products, Salt, Yellow Ochre	Frankincense	
SKIN PROBLEMS: Barley, Frankincense, *djaret*, Salt		
HAIR PROBLEMS: Blood, Ink-Powder, Ladanum		
RESPIRATORY CONDITIONS: Cumin, Colocynth, Dates, Figs, Frankincense, Juniper, Milk, Sebesten		
URINARY PROBLEMS: Dates, Grapes, Gum, Rush-Nuts, Wheat, Yellow Ochre	Celery (or Calotropis) Figs, Carob	
IMPOTENCE or PRIAPISM: Carob, Juniper, Hyoscyamus, Oils, Pine, Salt, Watermelon	Flax	
UTERINE DISORDERS: Frankincense		
ANAL DISORDERS: Barley, Cumin, Dates, Figs, Juniper, Myrrh, Raisins, Salt	Colocynth Frankincense	*djaret*
DIARRHEA: Figs, Oils, Pine, Raisins, Sebesten, Silphium, Yellow Ochre	Ostrich Eggs	*djaret*
NEED FOR LAXATIVE: Dates, *djaret*, Figs, Pine, Salt, Sebesten, Senna	Colocynth	
"WORMS:" Colocynth, Dates, Silphium		

TABLE 8-B. Presumed active ingredients used in 10–20% or 20–40% of prescriptions recommended in the Ebers Papyrus for conditions clearly stated to be associated with *wḫdw* or "rose" (its meaning is entirely obscure), or with magic. (See Appendix for details of each drug.)

Ingredients Included in 10–20% of Recipes for each CLINICAL INDICATION:	***In 20–40%***
DISORDERS OF *wḫdw*, and "ROSE," in:	
Belly and Wounds: Acacia, Ammi, Balanites Oil, Colocynth, *djaret*, Figs, Myrrh, Salt, Sebesten, Sory	
Jugular and Cardiac Areas: Ammi, Carob, Dates, *djaret*, Frankincense, Juniper	Figs
MAGICAL OR DIVINE DISEASE OF THE BELLY: Carob, Dates, Manna, Myrtle, Natron, Pine, Rush-Nuts, Salt, Yeast	Ammi Coriander *djaret* Frankincense

arrheals, and perhaps as carminatives, even if the latter drug class is no longer recognized in modern medicine), some of those agents were used primarily in the treatment of nongastrointestinal symptoms, such as aloe for eye disease and colocynth for respiratory ailments. These are undoubtedly instances in which the *swnw* thought he was directing his drugs into the *metu* distributing system of the body for delivery elsewhere, regardless of their effects on the bowels.

For the disorders of the *metu* in Table 8-B, we have no good clues about the patient's symptoms or chief complaints. When an ancient Egyptian consulted the medical papyri, he would have needed to know only his patient's chief symptoms in order to select an appropriate remedy; he probably already understood the underlying pathology, for which he did not need a reference manual like the Hearst or Ebers papyri. Such diagnostic and therapeutic reasoning—and it is logical, even if unsupportable by modern physiological concepts—probably provided the roots of humoral pathology, as elaborated later by Greek and Roman physicians, that survived until it simply disappeared as an acceptable working

◀ **TABLE 8-A.** Presumed active ingredients used in 10–20%, 20–40%, or more than 40%, of prescriptions recommended in the Ebers Papyrus for each of several clearly organ-system-based symptom complexes. (See Appendix for details of each drug.)

hypothesis in the wake of the microbiological discoveries of the nineteenth century. Even today, traces of the *wḫdw* can be detected in televised ads that urge us to use laxatives to improve our outlook on life and our interpersonal relationships.

To treat

In summary, although we can now recognize the pharmacological properties of at least some ancient Egyptian remedies, properties (or simply effects) that the *swnw* himself may also have recognized, we still do not know the exact reasoning that led him to prescribe most of his drugs in individual cases. Much of it must lie in mythology and magic. Nor do we have any clues about the frequency with which he prescribed them, much less about their true therapeutic efficacy. Indeed, we have no good reason to believe that most of the drugs routinely prescribed by the *swnw* could have produced any substantial clinical improvement by themselves; even if some did have selective effects, such as moving the bowels, that are not beneficial therapeutic effects *per se* (save in people who are constipated). The major exceptions to this rather negative generalization are, of course, the wound ointments made with honey and malachite.

Thus, we must conclude that the few surviving medical papyri are compilations of drugs most of which probably entered the Egyptian materia medica as a result of earlier associations with shamanistic or other magical rituals and practices, or because, by producing clearcut effects on intestinal activity, they reinforced the concept of the *wḫdw*. Whenever a patient recovered after a physician had prescribed for him—and it is entirely possible that as many as 90 percent of patients did recover following treatment (except in the face of the most virulent epidemics)[30]—it was likely to have been the result of the body's usually efficient built-in defenses against many of its ills, rather than the result of the medicine's selective pharmacological properties. Still, both the patient and his *swnw* had every good reason to be satisfied with the medical skills of ancient Egypt.

POSTSCRIPTS FROM THE FUTURE

Several ancient Egyptian drugs were still being used in the nineteenth century by physicians in Europe and America, and a few, such as aloe and castor oil, survived into the twentieth century. Other Egyptian materials entered Western medical use only temporarily. For instance, in the first century A.D., Dioscorides included many drugs that were indigenous to Egypt in his pioneering herbal, including papyrus:

> *It is of singular use in Physick for the unstopping of the mouth of ye Fistulas, being prepared, that is [,] being macerated in somme liquor & a linnen thread being tyed about it till it be drie. For being thus strengthened and put in, it is filled with moisture, and swelling, it opens the Fistulas . . . But ye Papyrus being burnt until the turning of it into ashes doth restrain the fretting ulcers in the mouth & everie part. But burnt paper doth doe this better.*[31]

Far more bizzare, to modern sensibilities at least—and certainly unthinkable to ancient Egyptians—was the use of mummies themselves as medicine, a fad that peaked in the seventeenth century. The rationale in this case was quite simple: mummies were tangible symbols of longevity. Sir Thomas Browne (1605–1682) noted that bits and pieces of mummy were recommended by contemporary physicians for treating epilepsy and gout, or to either enhance or inhibit blood clotting, or, by the French king Francis I, as a panacea. Although it is likely that much of the "mummy" of pharmaceutical commerce was only resin of unverifiable provenance, Browne's attack on the practice was eloquently cynical:

> *The Egyptian Mummies, which Cambyses or time hath spared, avarice now consumeth. Mummie is become Merchandise, Mizraim cures wounds, and Pharaoh is sold for balsams. In vain do individuals hope for immortality, or any patent from Oblivion. . . .*
>
> *Shall Egypt lend out her ancients unto chirurgeons and apothecaries, and Cheops and Psammiticus be weighed unto us for drugs? Shall we eat of Chamnes and Amoses in electuaries and pills, and be cured by cannibal mixtures? Surely such diet is dismal vampirism.*[32]

Physicians of the Enlightenment gave Egypt credit—implicitly at least—for their Unguentum Egyptiacum. It was made by boiling honey, verdegris (which was chiefly cupric acetate), and strong vinegar until the mixture became viscous and turned purple. The ancient *swnw* would have approved of the way in which, in 1794, this mixture was used by the physicians of Edinburgh, then probably the leading medical faculty in the Western world: "It is a very powerful application for cleansing and deterging foul [skin] ulcers, as well as for keeping down fungous flesh." However, the same physicians also thought that "these purposes may in general be answered by articles less acrid and exciting less pain," and that it was difficult to be sure of the unguent's true efficacy because some of the verdegris usually settled out while the medicine was being prepared.[33]

When Napoleon's army occupied Egypt in 1798, his medical staff judged the country to be surprisingly healthy, although smallpox and plague epidemics did break out from time to time. Dysentery accounted for much of the morbidity observed by the French, while respiratory diseases were uncommon. They saw malaria in some, but not all, cities, as well as ophthalmia, induced by blowing sand, not by micro-organisms. Finally, they thought that malnutrition and plague combined to negate the high birth rate of the capital city. Pierre Rouyer, a pharmacist attached to the scientific task force that accompanied the French army, listed the drugs sold in the apothecary shops of Cairo. Eighty-one of them (90 percent) were also found in the pharmacopoeias then current in France, and many were used regularly in Edinburgh and New England. A third of the eighteenth-century Egyptian drugs had been mentioned in the Ebers Papyrus; cathartics were especially prominent among them. Rouyer also noted that the physiological rationales for most of the drugs he catalogued were rooted in the ancient Hippocratic and Galenic humoral tradition. Thus, his study of drugs in Cairo's pharmacies reflects parallel developments in the medical therapeutics of the Mediterranean and Anglo-American worlds. Drugs that had first found use along the banks of the Nile in pharaonic times were still being used there in 1798, as well as by Europeans wherever they went. It seems most likely that Greco-Roman borrowings from ancient Egyptian usage had been preserved by Dioscorides and in medieval Arabic texts, and then transmitted to Renaissance Europe as well as back home to Islamic Egypt.[34]

In the early twentieth century, George Reisner listed, in the introduction to his edition of the hieratic text of the Hearst Papyrus, several household remedies of the Egyptians who worked at his excavations. These remedies seem to represent a virtually unbroken tradition since the days of the pharaohs:

1. For sore eyes, fresh dung of an ass, heated, laid on the eyes, and bound with a cloth.

2. For boils, the same.
3. For sore eyes, *ḥâra* weed boiled in water. Hold the eyes in the steam.
4. For headache, henna, dissolved in hot water and rubbed on forehead, temples and cheeks.
5. For pains in the stomach, leaves of wormwood (*šîḥ*) dried, rubbed to a powder and swallowed with a drink of water. . . .
7. For a wound, apply hot grease, or lime, or coffee grounds, or crushed onions.
8. To preserve the eyes of a child, drop them every day with verdegris dissolved in water.
9. To preserve the eyes of a man, rub the edges of the lids with *koḥl* (antimony).
10. For any ache or pain whatsoever, a charm may be obtained of one of the scribes skilled in charms. According to the scribe's directions, the charm is to be suspended [over] the affected part, or it is to be burnt and used as a fumigant.[35]

Dorothy Eady was an engaging twentieth-century English woman who lived for about 30 years at Abydos, the ancient holy place that had probably contributed to Imhotep's models for the Step Pyramid (see the Prologue). She had gone there in 1956, largely because it was the site of a great temple—perhaps the most truly beautiful in all Egypt—built by her personal idol, the pharaoh Seti I (1306–1290 B.C.). Eady quickly learned local medicinal lore; for instance, she used the sap and leaves of the sycomore fig to treat the rashes, burns, and other skin ailments of her fellow villagers. And she concluded that the water at the ruins of the even more ancient temple of Osiris nearby had healed some of her own ailments.[36]

Further striking evidence that certain practices of the *swnw* have survived into the late twentieth century emerges from a 1987 interview with a village *feki* ("magic man") conducted in Karima, Sudan, by Timothy Kendall of the Museum of Fine Arts, Boston.[37] Hussein Mustapha Ahmed, who was 47 years old, had achieved the highest rank among practitioners of folk medicine after studying as an apprentice to a friend's father for seven years, although most *feki* learn from their own fathers. Hussein, who was the first in his family to become one, said that his son would learn the profession "because he handles snakes and scorpions" —as did figures of Horus on many ancient healing statues.

Hussein was like the men Reisner described as "scribes skilled in charms." The modern *feki* attributed his own magical skills to his power over seven *jinn*, or genii, members of the vast hierarchy of supernatural beings who control everyday events. Among his professional tools were two magical stones that closely resembled special stones that had been excavated at ancient sites. But the mainstay of his business was composing *hijabs*, magical writings that consisted of verses of the Koran, the names of gods or archangels, or numbers arranged in patterns.

Some of these writings were designed to ward off unfriendly *jinns*, or even to cause death in a distant place. Hussein had recently written a spell for Kendall's cook to place around the neck of her chronically ill grandson, and another to keep a general in the Sudanese army from having a heart attack. Such *hijabs* were fairly expensive; the cook paid a week's wages—about six American dollars—for hers, while the general was charged a thousand dollars. Hussein could also provide spells, "so that a woman can have a baby, or so that she will be protected during pregnancy, or so that one will be protected against head wounds"—all are reminiscent of spells in the ancient papyri. He went on to point out that the ink of other *hijabs* could be washed off into water, thus transferring their power to the water—as had been recommended in some New Kingdom papyri.

Hussein carried a leather satchel filled with medicines for special purposes. Most appear to be long-term direct survivors from pharaonic Egypt:

> *Heart of baby crocodile. (Hussein placed small bits of it in* hijabs *designed to protect people from fear. Mixed with* nargin *wood oil it made a medicine a woman could rub on her husband's phallus to restore his potency.)*
>
> *Crocodile liver.*
>
> *Crocodile lung.*
>
> *Brain of baby. ("If the husband of a woman is 'not good,' she takes a little powder of this and puts it on her face, and her husband will come to her directly.")*
>
> *Saffron. ("You put this in water and you make a potion, and you drink it, and then you write in red ink that you will not have any illness. Then you never get sick.")*
>
> Dam el-Akhnein, *red coral from the Red Sea. ("You make the coral into a powder and you mix it with ground up cockscomb. Then you dry it, and put it in water for a child to drink, and this prevents bed-wetting.")*
>
> El-Karim, *a root. (Prevents sleep walking.)*
>
> *Dead bat. ("You grind up little pieces of this, mix them with sesame oil, and rub them on hives, and in three days you are cured.")*

Maya Sayel, *an incense. ("If you have a pain, you inhale the smoke of this and the pain will go away.")*

Pomegranate, which came in a little tin labelled as a remedy for scorpion bites, apparently purchased at a pharmacy. (Hussein said he applied it to scorpion stings after cutting the wound and sucking out the poison. "When I suck it out," he went on, "my mouth tingles from the poison. Then I apply this and say words.")

Sukar Nabat, *a sweet resin from a tree. ("If you get anything in your eye, you put this in your eye and it takes out the offending particle or ailment.")*

Hawa*("wind"), which Kendall thought was hashish. ("Use this, and the* jinn *come quickly.")*

Mughal azzrak, *a black seed. ("You burn it when a woman is three months pregnant, and it prevents miscarriage.")*

Hentib. *("If you have a toothache, you put this on your gums, and your tooth will come out.")*

Black cumin. ("If you have a constant headache, you smoke it as a cigarette.")

Mukhal azrak, *a white incense. ("This will bring lots of children to a woman.")*

Ambar kham, *little black pellets imported from India. ("If you have a 'snake' [tapeworm] in your stomach, you put one of these in your tea and drink it, and the 'snake' comes out.")*

Khedwe. *("If a woman eats one of these beans, she will not conceive for a year. If she eats ten of them, she will not conceive for ten years." When asked if he had had any complaints from dissatisfied customers, Hussein swore he had not. When asked about the source of these beans, he said "They come from a local tree, which I talk to.")*

Like Hussein, villagers in remote parts of Syria and Jordan exploit the *jinn* for healing purposes. They also rely on many of the same drugs the *swnw* used, such as honey, oil, plant remedies, animal products, and human milk, and, as the ancient Egyptians did, they place garlic in the vagina to determine if a woman is fertile (if she is, the odor of garlic will appear in her breath the next day). Also like the Egyptians, traditional practitioners of Arabic medicine believe that death cannot be postponed beyond its appointed time. However, unlike the *swnw*, Levantine healers use drugs, as well as cupping and bleeding techniques, derived explicitly from the humoral tradition.[38] Although it took shape chiefly in classical Greece, perhaps as a modification of the *swnw*'s ideas, humoralism was saved for the future in the writings of medieval Arabic physicians, like Rhazes, Avicenna, and Averroes, who transmitted the concept to both Western and Islamic medicine.

Some of Hussein's drugs appear in the Ebers and Hearst papyri. The ancient magical roots of the rationales behind virtually all of them are quite clear, even those we cannot be sure were prescribed by the *swnw*. But in this case, it is not the magical potency associated with the ancient past that seventeenth-century Europeans cited when prescribing remedies made with pieces of mummies, but the far more pragmatic (although fallacious) *post hoc, ergo propter hoc* association of recovery with its preceding treatment that accounts for Hussein's professional success in a village on the banks of the Nile in the late twentieth century.

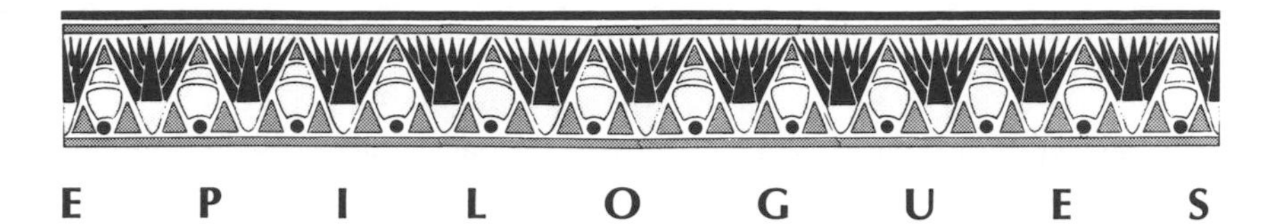

E P I L O G U E S

WHAT DIFFERENCE DID EGYPTIAN MEDICINE MAKE?

TO THE ANCIENT EGYPTIANS?

The spectrum of therapeutic choices available to the ancient Egyptians included a wide range of organic and inorganic materials on the one hand, and a variety of magico-religious procedures on the other. Although a few drugs may have provided some modest alleviation of symptoms, most therapeutic manoeuvres—magical or medicinal—could, at best, have provided only opportunities for wounds or illnesses to heal on their own. Indeed, many magical treatments were probably no less "effective" as cures than the drugs prescribed by the *swnw*, for the same reason. If so, then we cannot be too surprised that a substantial fraction of his remedies continued to be used by professional (and nonprofessional) healers in subsequent cultures, including our own. Save for a few infectious diseases, like trachoma and schistosomiasis, which were far more likely to be found in the Egyptian environment than in ours, the ancient physician's patients were subject to the same broad range of diseases and wounds that we are, even if most of them did not live long enough to develop the illnesses that afflict the elderly today. However, Egyptians may have been protected from some infections because ancient populations along the Nile were probably less dense than is necessary to maintain certain pathogenic microbes in human hosts, especially those bacteria and viruses that are most sensitive to the hot dry sun on the desert edge where most villages were built.

Summarizing the actual achievements of ancient physicians requires making some giant leaps, from the few demonstrable facts unearthed and first interpreted by scholars in the field to a number of later-generation inferences whose validities cannot be assessed rigorously. Compounding the difficulty, there are virtually no first-hand records of the actual clinical activities and successes of any of the *swnw* (with the possible exception of the Smith Papyrus). Nonetheless, if we take the few available clues at their collective face value, we can conclude that Egyptian physicians could exploit systematic methods for observing and categorizing the facts in their patients' cases, and that they used those facts to arrive at rational diagnostic, prognostic, and therapeutic decisions, even if it is uncertain whether more than a minority of the *swnw* used such a full range of intellectual skills. They did produce the first known medical texts, the first written observations of human anatomy (which were not very analytical in any case), the first surgical and drug therapies, the first splints and bandages, and the first medical vocabulary. The extent to which the Egyptians may have preceded the even older cultures of Mesopotamia in developing a medical "system" is arguable; the two cradles of civilization were in communication with each other at least by the early third millennium B.C. It would probably be more surprising if the Egyptians had *not* accomplished what they did in medicine.[1]

We are hard put to recognize "science," at least by today's definitions, among the professional practices or accomplishments of the *swnw*. John Wilson has noted that the Egyptians' "pragmatic nature in medicine and their fear of the gods prevented them from prying into matters which were not direct and useful," and that they showed little inclination toward change, much less for experimentation.[2] R. W. Sloley, who would have agreed, concluded that the Egyptians never had the consuming intellectual curiosity of the Greeks, their cultural successors across the Mediterranean,[3] while Warren R. Dawson went so far as to assert that the Egyptians "were incapable of . . . abstract thought,"[4] even if they did recognize the power of magic, which, along with the *wḫdw*, they accepted as proven fact.

It is almost certain that they did not perform controlled or comparative medical experiments like those demanded by today's scientific methodology, nor did the Egyptians employ physiological abstractions in any way related to ours. Nevertheless, they did develop what they regarded as expedient solutions to real health problems. George Sarton, who probably understood the word "science" better than most of its historians, thought that the pragmatic methodology of the *swnw* does illustrate the scientific process, even if the illustration is a pale one that shines brightly only in the Smith Papyrus.[5] Sarton, Owsei Temkin, and Hermann Ranke have concluded that Egyptian medicine flowered as a "science" only during the Old Kingdom. They suggest that over succeeding centuries medical science, such as it was, became diluted, confused, and forced to accept religious impositions during the foreign conquests and internal disorders of the Intermediate Periods preceding the Middle and New Kingdoms, and again during the late New Kingdom. The dilution process was accelerated by the ascent of the priestly caste to temporal power during the first millennium B.C. From the New Kingdom on, the modern scholars have argued, medicine seems to have degenerated to include increasing proportions of magical practices as Egypt's more material culture, typified by the dazzling contents of Tutankamen's tomb, approached its most flamboyant zenith.[6]

It would seem highly unlikely that the professional skills of the *swnw* were sufficient to alter substantially either the health patterns of the Egyptian population or of their individual patients. Their laxative drugs probably did move their patients' bowels (at least when given by mouth), and their wound dressings probably did control infectious organisms long enough to permit some wounds to heal satisfactorily. Their attempts to reduce dislocations and simple fractures undoubtedly benefitted some of those patients. But by and large, we can only conclude that, at their best, the ancient physician's efforts merely permitted nature to complete her usual healing course; for the most serious problems neither the *swnw*, as he may have known, nor nature could furnish definitive solutions.[7]

TO LATER CIVILIZATIONS?

Beginning in the seventh century B.C., the Greeks' trading colonies in Egypt permitted them to absorb what they wished from the culture of the pharaohs, whose native-ruled dynasties were already disappearing,[8] even if the medical remnants of the older culture were not as scientific in quality as the Greeks would come to consider essential. The way toward modern medicine still had a long way to go: Hippocrates, our own "father of medicine," antedated us by about as many centuries as Imhotep antedated him.[9]

Like Herodotus, Homer remarked on the Egyptians' reputation for healing, especially for the remedies they made from plants that grew along the Nile. According to the *Odyssey* (probably composed in the eighth century B.C., contemporary with Dynasties XXIII–XXIV), one night Queen Helen of Sparta dosed her banquet guests with a drug that could assuage their painful memories of the Trojan War:

> *This powerful anodyne was one of many useful drugs which had been given to the daughter of Zeus [i.e., Helen] by an Egyptian lady, Polydamna, the wife of Thon [i.e., the god Seth]. For the fertile soil of Egypt is most rich in herbs, many of which are wholesome in solution, though many are poisonous. And in medical knowledge the Egyptian leaves the rest of the world behind. He is a true son of Paeeon the Healer.*[10]

We have seen in Chapter One that foreign monarchs sometimes imported Egyptian physicians for their courts. Later, as Egypt became part of the Persian, Hellenistic, and then the Roman empires, her international contacts throughout the world increased. Both normal trade connections and the great Greek research center at Alexandria provided direct potential pathways for the transmission of Egyptian medical thought to the rest of the ancient world, just as some Egyptian religious practices penetrated to the geographical limits of that world, and thence into more modern times.[11]

Many Egyptian medical terms and practices were adopted by the Hebrews; their word *rofe'im* is equivalent to *swnw*.[12] From the Egyptians the Greeks probably derived several pathophysiological concepts which re-emerged much later with the effects of the *wḫdw* refined and transmuted into the humoral assumptions of Hippocrates and Galen, although this point is still debated. For instance, the Greeks' concept of pathogenic digestive residues (*perittoma*)[13] is surely closely related to the *wḫdw*, even if the two concepts are not identical. The transfer, if it did occur, was probably facilitated by the absence of experimental methods, in either culture, for *testing* the underlying premises.

Other more practical, or more trivial, medical techniques that migrated to Greece included several medicinal plants, the structure of drug prescriptions, the practices of prenatal prognosis and gynecological fumigations, the concept of "defluxions," and the healing value of temple sleep ("incubation").[14] Despite assertions to the contrary,[15] it was not the Hippocratic authors who first recognized nature's power to heal spontaneously without professional medical intervention; the Old Kingdom *swnw* who recommended that certain patients be "left at their mooring stakes" was a far earlier advocate of the *vis medicatrix naturae* (the "healing power of nature"). Parallels and derivations from the Egyptian medical papyri appear in Arab medical compilations of the seventh through ninth centuries A.D., and in medieval medical manuscripts; not all were transmitted solely through Dioscorides.[16] Some drugs from the Nile valley could still be found in European and American pharmacology and pharmacognosy texts in the seventeenth to twentieth centuries.[17] Imhotep even appears as an alchemist ("Senior Philosophus") in a sixteenth-century woodcut illustrating a tenth-century Arab manuscript.[18] That the *wḫdw* was still alive and well in colonial Boston is clearly evident in Dr. John Perkins' note that "Purges are chiefly to prevent any putrid matter from entering the habit."[19] The ancient *swnw* could not have foretold it, but they had produced the embryo of one of the world's fittest traditions.

TO IMHOTEP?

Among the Greeks' trophies from the period of their closest intercourse with Egypt was Imhotep himself. Over the two millennia after his death, his reputation grew until he finally came to be regarded as the Egyptian god of medicine. When the Greeks arrived, they identified and assimilated him (as Imouthes, the Greek version of his name) with their own recently appointed medical deity, Asklepios.[20]

Imhotep must have been held in exceptionally high esteem throughout the history of ancient Egypt, a sort of national historic treasure. Only two or three men other than pharaohs—who sometimes functioned as gods in many of their official capacities even while they were in this world—ever achieved formal deification. As early as the first years of the New Kingdom, during a brief renaissance of the art styles of the Old Kingdom, scribes made pilgrimages to the fountainhead of that style, the Step Pyramid, and dropped miniature libations to Imhotep on their ink palettes. But long before then, a new religious cult had begun to develop around his memory, a cult that would survive into the Christian era.[21]

One document (Oxyrhynchus Papyrus 1381) suggests that Imhotep had been worshipped as early as a century after his death, although the story seems to have been concocted in the second century A.D., perhaps to bolster the traditional rights of his priests. Nevertheless, the key episode in the text graphically illustrates healing by incubation with Imhotep as the "hero":

> *It was night, when every living creature was asleep except those in pain, but divinity showed itself the more effectively; a violent fever*

burned me, and I was convulsed with loss of breath and coughing, owing to the pain proceeding from my side. Heavy in the head with my troubles I was lapsing half-conscious into sleep [at a temple, probably that of Imhotep at Memphis], and my mother, as a mother would for her child [although the patient had earlier described himself as aged], . . . was sitting without enjoying even a short period of slumber, when suddenly she perceived—it was no dream or sleep, for her eyes were open immovably, though not seeing clearly, for a divine and terrifying vision came to her, easily preventing her from observing the god himself or his servants, whichever it was. In any case there was some one whose height was more than human, clothed in shining raiment and carrying in his left hand a book, who after merely regarding me two or three times from head to foot disappeared. When she had recovered herself, she tried, still trembling, to wake me, and finding that the fever had left me and that much sweat was pouring off me, did reverence to the manifestation of the god, and then wiped me and made me more collected . . . everything that she saw in the vision appeared to me in dreams. After these pains in my side had ceased and the god had given me yet another assuaging cure, I proclaimed his benefits. [This was not enough for the god, and he forced the writer to return to an earlier promise to write a book about the god and his cult, because] a written record is an undying [reward] of gratitude, from time to time renewing its youth in the memory. Every Greek tongue will tell thy story, and every Greek man will worship the son of Ptah, Imouthes [i.e., Imhotep/Asklepios].[22]

Because of his contributions to Egypt's collective national memory (and perhaps because of other factors we may never be able to identify), Imhotep's tomb seems to have become a tourist attraction shortly after it was built. Its precise location has never been identified satisfactorily, although it was probably at Sakkara, the necropolis of Memphis. When, during the reign of Ptolemy II Philadelphus (285–246 B.C.), Manetho came to write his history of Egypt, he noted that Imhotep "reckoned [with] the Egyptians as Asklepios [with the Greeks] on account of his medical skill, and who invented building with hewn stone; he also devoted attention to writing." Granite flooring had been used at Sakkara as early as Dynasty I, for the cenotaph of the fifth king, Usaphais (also known as Den, he died about 2900 B.C.), and limestone was used to build the first known stone walls, those of the Dynasty II tomb of Zoser's close predecessor, Khasekhemui (d. ca. 2649 B.C.); both he and his father may have built small stone temples as well. However, the tomb was below ground, and the temples are long gone. Thus, the Step Pyramid complex remains to this day the principal evidence for awarding to Imhotep all claims of priority for building in stone on a monumental scale.[23] The ancient Egyptians' reverence for his pioneering accomplishments further underscores those claims.

For many centuries Imhotep was regarded as a "demi-god," a status sufficiently important to warrant the widespread manufacture of small statues showing him as a scribe. At least 400 have been preserved. In these figures he is seated, holding a papyrus scroll on his lap wearing a skull cap and a pleated skirt (see Figure 2). The symbol of a man reading had long been used to represent wisdom and divine inspiration. Some statuettes portray him with pectoral jewelry, but never with the full trappings of deity. Fragmentary evidence suggests that Imhotep may have been worshipped as early as Dynasty IV, and that the Egyptians became more interested in healing gods during the New Kingdom, perhaps as they became more uncertain about the afterlife. Then sometime after Cambyses' conquest of Egypt in 525 B.C., Imhotep begins to appear in inscriptions and papyri as a full-fledged god. His formal apotheosis may have occurred during a second Old Kingdom renaissance that began during the immediately preceding native dynasty (Dynasty XXVI), when Egyptians looked back to their new god's architectural innovations at Sakkara with pride and admiration. Dignitaries of the Late Dynastic Period (Dynasties XXV through XXX, 712–332 B.C.) even sought to be buried near the Step Pyramid because they regarded Imhotep as a fountainhead of Egyptian culture.[24]

Remembering that Zoser's vizier had never practiced the healing arts during his lifetime, we must ask how he came to be chosen as the Egyptians' god of medicine. One factor leading to the choice of Imhotep to fill that niche must simply have been that the Egyptians had never had such a deity on a full-time basis before. Perhaps their ancestors, whose traditional gods probably originated as animal/clan totems in the Predynastic era, had felt no special need for a god of medicine, or perhaps it was merely an oversight. It may also be that the *swnw* had developed a sufficiently strong sense of professional self-identification by the sixth century B.C. that they finally came to feel they deserved their own divine patron. By then the priestly caste had assumed even more importance in Egyptian life than it had in the past; presumably the priest-healers shared the same spotlight. Neither the *swnw* nor the healing priests had ever had their own special deity, one on a par with the gods whom the priests served even before they served their patients. Thus, perhaps the healing profession needed a god of medicine as a status symbol, especially if physicians were becoming more important to a population that had become increasingly skeptical about what happened after death.

Imhotep's deification may also have been facilitated by his links with Thoth, who was revered as the scribe of the gods and the inventor of all the arts and sciences—a sort of part-time god of medicine. Many thousands of mummified ibises—which were associated with Thoth—were buried in vast underground chambers at Sakkara during the Late Period.[25] But the strongest links between him and Imhotep were probably forged from the traditionally dominant role of scribes in Egyptian life, as is clearly implied in the many statues of Imhotep made before his final apotheosis that show him as a scribe. Adolf Erman noted that the Egyptians had a "mania for writing,"[26] the skill that distinguished the scribal profession from all others. Long before she took up nursing, Florence Nightingale summarized the Egyptians' appreciation of learning and books: "There is something very beautiful in all knowledge being so religious that the very professing of it consecrated a man. To the Egyptians Sir Isaac Newton would have been as holy as St. Augustine; the one kind of knowledge was as much inspiration as the other."[27] Her comparison was apt, if a bit effusive.

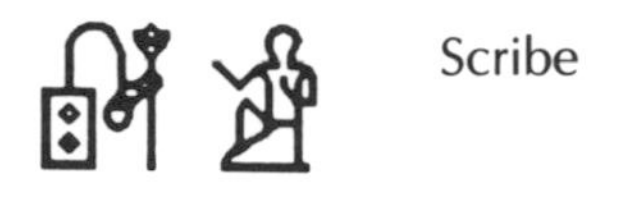

Scribes assumed increasingly important roles as calculators, in business and in levying taxes, during Dynasties XIX and XX, and their ranks increased significantly. By then, the theocratic state had come to be so dominated by clerks acting for the pharaoh and the land-owning temples that the scribes were seen as the people chiefly responsible for maintaining the country's collective prosperity. During the Old Kingdom, Egyptians had been somewhat individualistic, but under the New Kingdom they became increasingly nationalistic and communal, bringing into their lives a new emphasis on ritual and on conformity to the common cause.[28] Scribes were, of course, highly visible at tax-collection time, which probably epitomized the common cause of both the villagers and their king.

Finally, although Egyptians had an extraordinarily high regard for the scribes' learning,[29] it was not solely because learning was its own reward—despite Miss Nightingale's hyperbole. Rather, it was because the scribe was independent of virtually all other members of Egyptian society, while most of the population was accountable directly to him, especially when it was time to pay taxes. A school exercise book written during Dynasty XX (1196–1070 B.C.) emphasizes the personal benefits of the learned professions: "Writing is more enjoyable than enjoying a basket of [?] and beans; more enjoyable than a mother's giving birth, when her heart knows no distaste. . . . Happy is the heart [of] him who writes; he is young each day."[30]

More to the point was another copybook exercise that seems to have been composed during the Middle Kingdom and then recopied by many generations of student scribes at least until the end of the New Kingdom. It is now called "The Satire of the Trades" because it caricatures the disincentives to the most common occupations along the Nile—heavy labor, unhealthy work conditions, insect bites, fatigue, and dirt—even if reliefs and other texts show that Egyptians took pride in their field work and artisanry. The "Satire" focusses, perhaps with tongue in cheek, on the material benefits of being able to write:

I have seen many beatings—
Set your heart on books!
I watched those seized for labor—
There's nothing better than books!
. . . . .
I'll make you love scribedom more than your mother,
I'll make its beauties stand before you;
It's the greatest of all callings,
There's none like it in the land.
. . . . .
See, there's no profession without a boss,
Except for the scribe; he is the boss.
Hence if you know writing,
It will do better for you
Than those professions I've set before you,
Each more wretched than the other.
. . . . .
Lo, no scribe is short of food
And of riches from the palace.[31]

In 1817 Percy Bysshe Shelley used a fragmented colossus of Ramesses II near the necropolis at Thebes to dramatize the plight of "Ozymandias, king of kings," as he pleaded, "Look on my works, ye mighty, and despair!" In his case, according to the Romantic poet, it was not the pharaoh's power and empire that had survived, but the work of the sculptor—the artist. In the case of Imhotep, it was not even his architectural innovations but his wisdom, reflected in his books, that was used in the same way in Papyrus Chester Beatty IV (now in the British Museum) to illustrate the true sources of immortality—in the minds of men:

[The first scribes in history] made heirs for themselves of books,
Of Instructions they had composed.
They gave themselves [the scroll] as lector-priest
The writing-board as loving son [i.e., the person who maintained the funerary cult].
Instructions [i.e., their writings] are their tombs,
The reed pen is their child,
The stone-surface their wife.
People great and small
Are given them as children,
For the scribe, he is their leader.

Their portals and mansions have crumbled,
Their ka-servants are [gone];
Their tombstones are covered with soil,
Their graves are forgotten.
. . . . .

Man decays, his corpse is dust,
All his kin have perished;
But a book makes him remembered
Through the mouth of its reciter.
Better is a book than a well-built house,
Than tomb-chapels in the west;
. . . . .
Is there one here like Hardedef? [Cheops' son, regarded as another Old Kingdom sage]
Is there another like Imhotep?
. . . . .
Death made their names forgotten
But books made them remembered![32]

A good education even seems to have paved the way to "greater happiness and success" in the army.[33] Thus, it is not hard to imagine the

Old Kingdom vizier, whose reputation for wisdom had survived for 2500 years, being chosen to be the noncontroversial representative of the healing arts because, as writing and medical skills had long gone hand in hand, so had they been personified together in Thoth.

Once deified (through whatever chain of sacerdotal or political reasoning), Imhotep naturally required divine parents. For his father, the Egyptians gave him Ptah, the primeval god of the Old Kingdom capital at Memphis, near the new god's famous Step Pyramid. Sekhmet, the lion-headed goddess of war and disease whose priests had long doubled as healers, became Imhotep's divine mother. Even his earthly mother, Kherednankh, and his wife, Ronpe-nofret, were elevated into the auxiliary pantheon. In time, Ptah, Sekhmet, and Imhotep came to be worshipped as an especially holy Triad of Memphis, and finally Imhotep came to rival even the "*immensa Ptah*" of Verdi's *Aida* in northern Egypt.[34]

After his apotheosis Imhotep was portrayed, according to custom, holding the *ankh*, the life-symbol shown only in the hands of gods. He was given no other special divine insignia except, sometimes, a scepter or wand to signify his elevation to the godhead. Because he was reputed to have designed the first temple of Horus at Edfu, a little south of Thebes, a Ptolemaic relief of him there shows Imhotep holding a scroll and clothed in a leopard skin, but the latter was an insignia of priesthood, not of divinity. Elsewhere in the temple, he is called a "great god, residing at Edfu, at whose order everybody lives, who cures any illness in Egypt." When Coptic Christians occupied the temple, they obliterated his face from the relief, as they did all the "pagan" gods.[35]

Over the centuries Imhotep acquired his own temples. The largest and most famous was at Memphis; the Greeks called it the Asklepion. Its chief priestesses, who had to be twin sisters, presided each year over six celebrations of major events in the god's career, beginning with his birth, continuing through his death, and culminating in his apotheosis. One of the most famous of late Egyptian sanctuaries, it may have been built on the supposed (or even actual) site of his tomb. The temple was destroyed in 380 A.D. on orders of the Christian Roman emperor Theodosius during a surfeit of missionary zeal.[36]

Smaller shrines to Imhotep were built at the mortuary temple of Rameses III at Medinet Habu, near the Valley of Kings, and at the temple of Ptah at Thebes (now part of the Karnak temple complex at Luxor). A Greek named Polyaratus wrote that a visit to one of these two Theban shrines to Imhotep cured him of a complaint that had bothered him for eight years.[37] The new deity was also venerated at two small Ptolemaic shrines on the upper terrace of Queen Hatshepsut's spectacular mortuary

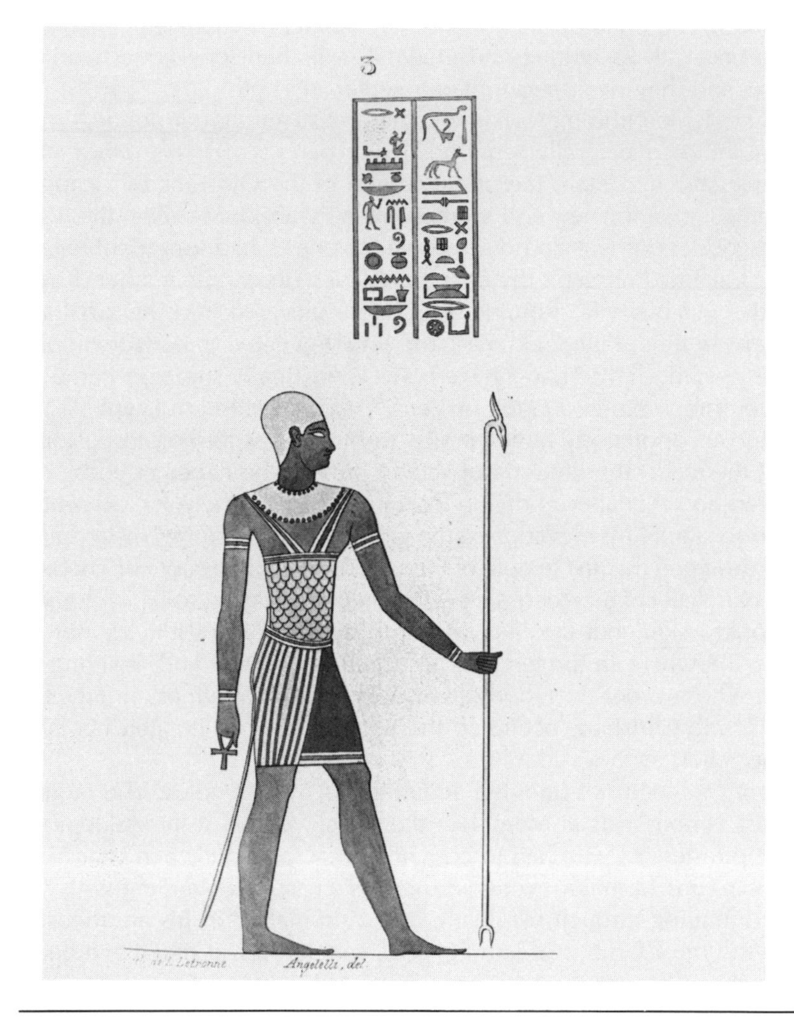

FIGURE 18. Drawing of a relief portraying Imhotep as a god, from his temple at Philae. He holds an *ankh* in his right hand and a god's scepter in his left. From Jean François Champollion, *Momunents de l'Égypte et de la Nubie* (Paris, 1835-45), vol. 1, plate 78.

temple at nearby Deir-el-Bahri; a Greek physician carved graffiti commemorating his visit there in the second century A.D. And there the god Imhotep is said to have appeared in a dream that resulted in the cure of two infertile patients. Similarly, Ptolemy V Epiphanes (205–180 B.C.) erected a small temple to Imhotep that abutted the imposing temple of Isis on the island of Philae at the first cataract of the Nile. The new shrine commemorated the birth of a royal son (who became Ptolemy VI Philometor) as a direct result of appeals to Imhotep after seven years of childless marriage. The story is reminiscent of the anachronistic tale of King Zoser and the ancient famine (see Chapter Two) that had been carved on the nearby island of Sehel not long before Ptolemy V built his temple. In 550 A.D. Ptolemy's temple, too, was deactivated by a Roman emperor, Justinian, but it can still be visited today, now that the temples on Philae that were under water for six months each year (after the sluices of the first Aswan dam went into operation in 1902) have been moved to a nearby higher island called Agilka.[38]

Another tale of pregnancy resulting from incubation was inscribed during the reign of Cleopatra VII (51–30 B.C.) on a funerary stele found at Memphis (British Museum no. 147). The deceased was a 30-year-old woman named Taimhotep who, at the age of 14, had married a high priest of Ptah at Memphis:

> *I was pregnant by [my husband] three times but did not bear a male child, only three daughters. I prayed together with the high priest to the majesty of the god great in wonders, effective in deeds, who gives a son to him who has none: Imhotep Son of Ptah.*
>
> *He heard our pleas, he hearkened to his prayers. The majesty of this god came to the head of the high priest in a revelation. He said, "Let a great work be done in the holy of holies of Ankhtawi, the place where my body is hidden. As reward for it I shall give you a male child."*
>
> *When [my husband] awakened from this he kissed the ground to the august god . . . He performed the opening of the mouth for the august god. He made a great sacrifice of all good things . . . In return [the god] made me conceive a male child.*
>
> *He was born . . . on the Offering-feast of the august god Imhotep Son of Ptah. [The child's] appearance was like that of [Imhotep]. There was jubilation over him by the people of Memphis. He was given the name of Imhotep . . . Everyone rejoiced over him.*[39]

The cult of Imhotep achieved its widest popularity during the Roman occupation of Egypt. By that time he was extolled as providing the country with both foreign treasure and the Nile's treasure, fertility, and even as guaranteeing the political and cosmic order. A long hymn to Imhotep as a kind-hearted (albeit somewhat junior) god was inscribed on a doorpost of the temple of Ptah at Karnak, probably during the reign of the emperor Tiberius (14–37 A.D.).[40] A few years later, the emperor Claudius (41–54 A.D.) caused the wall of the temple of the cow-eared goddess Hathor at Dendera to be decorated with a lengthy "Veneration of Imhotep" overlooking the sanatorium that provided magically treated water for the cure of the ill:

> *Praise to you, O god, borne a god, divine offspring of Ptah . . . O Imhotep . . . who restores what is destroyed everywhere in the temples, of perfect intelligence, who calculates everything, skillful like [Thoth], the great . . . successful in his activities, who knows the prescriptions and the recipes, which are written upon his heart, who lets be known the movement of the stars . . . who attenuates famine, skillful in his words, experienced in the divine writings, who gives life to the people and protects the pregnant, who gets the sterile with child, who gives a son to everyone who implores it, who protects the child, who regenerates the age of those who serve god, who soothes illness.*
>
> *Great wonderful appearance which stays on earth; there are no troubles as long as he is to be seen every day. Your secret appearance is great in towns and nomes; your throne is high in the houses of the gods in the Two Lands. They rejoice if they see you hearing the prayers of everybody.*[41]

This paean summarizes and epitomizes both the myths and the verifiable records, at least insofar as records were available then, pertaining to the life and deification of Imhotep as the quintessential ancient intellectual.

His effective lifespan was, then, somewhat longer than that of his country's native civilization or of her medical tradition, from his birth to the final extinction of his cult before the zealous onslaught of piously unforgiving Christianity. Imhotep's architectural accomplishments are very real; they initiated the tradition of building in stone that survives, however attenuated, even today. Cyril Aldred even credits him with having created "Egyptian high culture."[42] Very late Egyptian texts that refer to Imhotep provide tantalizing windows on several medical beliefs of the time, but Zoser's vizier has left us a paradox: he was, literally, the first physician to be worshipped on a pedestal, although there is no good evidence that he ever practiced any of the healing arts—at least, not before he became a god.

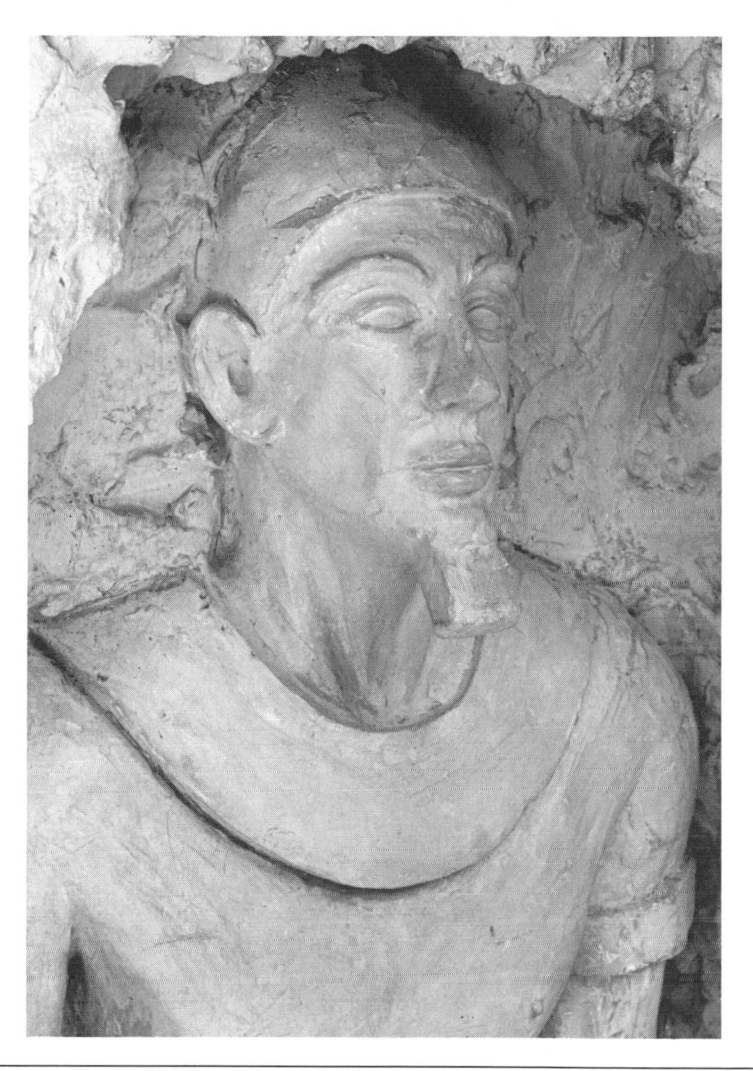

FIGURE 19. An example of modern medical veneration of Imhotep, based on Osler's 1923 description of him as "the first figure of a physician to stand out clearly from the mists of antiquity." Detail of a statue conceived and executed between 1939 and 1954 by Doris Appel for her Hall of Medicine sculptures for the Medical Museum of the Armed Forces Institute of Pathology in Washington, D.C., and now at the Boston University School of Medicine. (Photograph courtesy Fred Delorey)

A POSTSCRIPT FROM NINETEENTH-CENTURY BOSTON

If it was the first god of medicine who invented the prototype of the world's grandest funerary monument, it is fitting that one of America's most distinguished physicians invented today's landscaped cemetery, coupling it with new techniques for lasting and sanitary burial practices. Dr. Jacob Bigelow (1786–1879) of Boston was already famous for his contributions to American medical botany and pharmaceutical standardization when, in 1825, he conceived the idea that culminated in the opening of the Mount Auburn Cemetery across the Charles River in Cambridge six years later. Not only had he become interested in the Egyptians' methods for preserving their dead from decomposition, he also incorporated Egyptian decorative motifs into his plans for the new cemetery.[43]

Dr. Bigelow designed its entrance gate as an echo of examples he had seen in pictures of the great temples at Dendera and Karnak. He

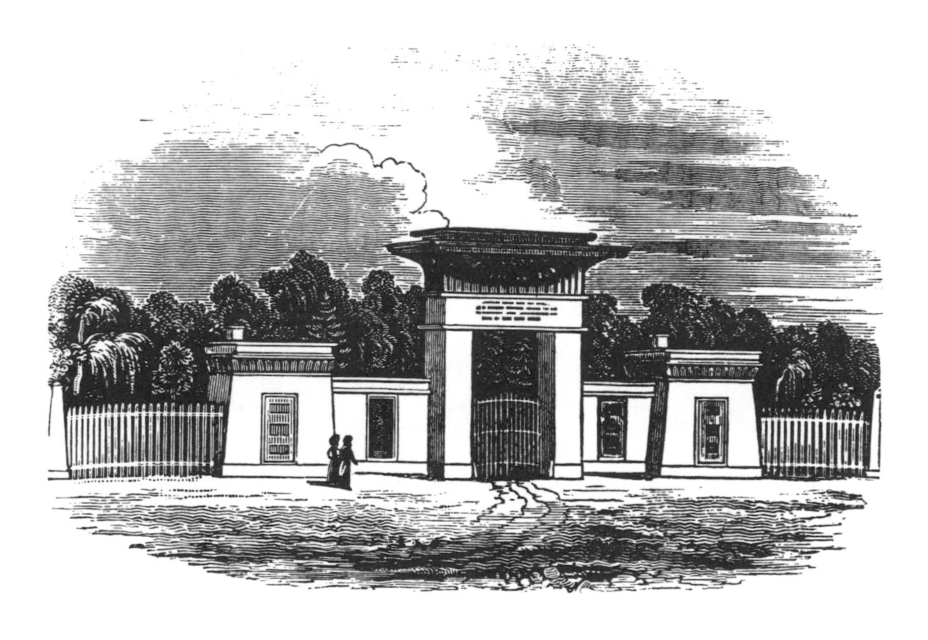

FIGURE 20. Entrance to Mount Auburn Cemetery, Cambridge, Massachusetts, from *The Picturesque Pocket Companion and Visitor's Guide through Mount Auburn* (Boston, 1839). (Courtesy, Boston Medical Library).

encouraged families to commission gravestones shaped like miniature Egyptian obelisks, and at least one tomb hollowed into a hillside at Mt. Auburn has a façade like that of an idealized miniature Egyptian temple. After the Civil War, he commissioned, from the noted American sculptor Martin Milmore (1844–1883), a large sphinx to memorialize those who had died in the war. At the unveiling ceremony in 1872, Bigelow, who was almost totally blind by then, remarked that the sphinx at the great pharaonic necropolis at Giza was the "most stupendous work of sculpture which the world has seen." He was familiar with the engravings published by the early explorers and archeologists, and with the sights his son had seen when visiting Egypt. The donor of the sculpture closed his dedicatory remarks by pointing out that he had chosen a sphinx to memorialize a tragic war in the imaginative necropolis he had designed 40 years earlier because the lion body symbolized power, while the female human face (a Greek substitute for the classical Egyptian male face) represented beauty and peace.

Bigelow's architectural innovation flourished immediately. The Granary Burying Ground on Boston's Tremont Street, where Paul Revere and other heroes of the American Revolution are enshrined in what had begun as a Puritan cemetery decorated with death's heads, crossbones, and cherubic promises of the life to come, was modernized in 1841 with a gateway derived from one at Karnak, the most monumental temple ever built. But one now barely notices the incongruity that Dr. Bigelow's innovation prompted on that grey downtown corner of Boston. A massive Egyptian gate provides entry to a veritable forest of obelisks in New Haven's Grove Street Cemetery. A small Egyptian-style temple was erected in the Lowell, Massachusetts, cemetery in 1890 as a mausoleum for an eight-year-old boy who had died five years earlier. More peculiarly, simplified versions of an Egyptian temple gate surround the base of the awkwardly truncated obelisk that commemorates Andrew Jackson's victory in the Battle of New Orleans.

It is pleasing, I think, to contemplate the two distinguished figures in the healing arts who invented new ways of memorializing the dead, both using motifs from the banks of the Nile. The chief difference between Bigelow and Imhotep was, of course, that only one was truly a professional healer; the other was only a god.

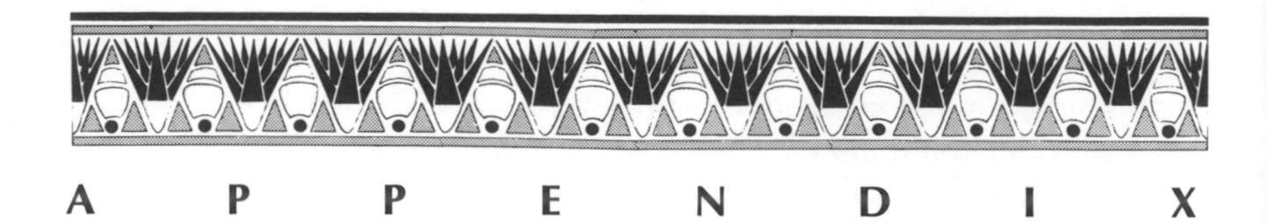

A P P E N D I X

THE MATERIA MEDICA OF PHARAONIC EGYPT

INTRODUCTION

This glossary of drug substances used in ancient Egyptian remedies (but excluding those associated with explicitly magical operations) is based chiefly on Ebbell's translation and interpretation of the Ebers Papyrus, supplemented by other sources cited below. Some identifications may not be completely accurate by all taxonomic standards, but this synthesis of others' scholarship probably represents the most that can be accomplished in the absence of an Egyptian textbook of botany based on Linnaean concepts.

This Appendix has been designed chiefly as a guide to the kinds of drug ingredients that ancient Egyptians employed in treating their sick, and some of the reasons they were prescribed. It cannot be assumed, much less proved, that any of these materials truly benefitted the *swnw*'s patients, nor can they be assumed to be effective therapies today. As noted in Chapter Five, the *swnw* seems not to have capitalized thoroughly on even the clearly evident pharmacological properties of some of his common remedies, while he expected more from others than they could possibly have delivered. However, as shown in Chapter Three, two ingredients—honey and copper salts—might well have been effective inhibitors of bacterial growth on wound surfaces.

The Ebers Papyrus gives 842 prescriptions, or drug recipes, that are not explicitly magical. They are made from about 328 different ingredients; of these, 197 (60.1 percent), in addition to the mysterious *djaret*, have not been translated, but they account for only 16.8 percent of all 3552 separate mentions of individual ingredients. The recipes contain an average of 4.2 ingredients each.

For each entry in CAPITAL LETTERS, the following information is given, as available:

1. *Ebbell's translation* (or, if he left it untranslated, a more recent one), *followed by the most likely biological, chemical, or mineralogical identification of the substance*. A question mark within parentheses (?) indicates that Ebbell was unsure of his translation and that no better identification has yet appeared. An asterisk (*) indicates that the drug was commonly sold in Cairo's apothecary shops as late as 1798. Entries in lower case are materials mentioned in other medical papyri or are synonyms for entries given in upper case.
2. *The fraction, in percent, of the 842 Ebers Papyrus prescriptions which include each drug material*. Entries with no incidence values are materials not mentioned in the Ebers Papyrus but which were in the list compiled by Leake from the Hearst and other medical papyri, or in the Chester Beatty VI Papyrus (which gives 41 remedies for afflictions of the anus).
3. *Clinical indications for use of the material in ancient Egypt*. These conclusions are based on tabulations of the frequencies with which the author of the Ebers Papyrus recommended them for use in diseases of various organ systems, including the *metu* (and *wḫdw* within the *metu*). That is, if a substantial majority of the clinical indications for any one drug material was concentrated in any one anatomic area, I could conclude that the material was used relatively selectively for those indications; or, if the recommendations covered many or most disease categories, I concluded that the material was used relatively non-selectively.
4. *Modern concepts of each drug ingredient's pharmacological or therapeutic properties, if any*, are given in square brackets [ ]. Modern concepts of these drugs' actions often bear little or no resemblance to the *swnw*'s use of them, and some of the "modern" concepts included here have been abandoned as concepts of drug efficacy have altered over the past half century or so.

SOURCES: B. Ebbell, trans., *The Papyrus Ebers: the Greatest Egyptian Medical Document* (Copenhagen, 1937); Chauncey D. Leake, *The Old Egyptian Medical Papyri* (Lawrence, Kans., 1952); Frans Jonckheere, *Le Papyrus Médical Chester Beatty* (Brussels, 1947); Loufty Boulos, *Medicinal Plants of North Africa* (Algonac, Mich., 1983); Alfred Lucas, *Ancient Egyptian Materials and Industries*, 4th ed., rev. by J. R. Harris (London, 1962); Warren R. Dawson, "Studies in the Egyptian Medical Texts," *Journal of Egyptian Archaeology 18* (1932): 150–154; *19* (1933): 133–137; *20* (1934): 41–46, 185–188; *21* (1935): 37–40; Edward Brovarski, Susan K. Doll, and Rita E. Freed, eds., *Egypt's Golden Age: the Art of Living in the New Kingdom, 1558–1085 B.C.* (Boston, 1982); William J. Darby, Paul Ghalioungui, and Louis Grivetti, *Food: the Gift of Osiris*, 2 vols. (New York, 1977); Dimitri Meeks, *Année Lexicographique*, 3 vols. (Paris: 1980–1982); Johanna Dittmar, *Blumen und Blumensträuse als Opfergabe im Alten Ägypten* (Berlin, 1986); Sue D'Auria, Peter Lacovara, and Catherine H. Roehrig, eds., *Mummies and Magic: the Funerary Arts of Ancient Egypt* (Boston, 1988).

Later uses of many of the drugs listed in this glossary may be found in some detail in: Robert T. Gunther, ed., *The Greek Herbal of Dioscorides* (Oxford, 1934), although we still await a definitive English translation; John M. Riddle, *Dioscorides on Pharmacy and Medicine* (Austin, Texas, 1985); Martin Levey, trans., *The Medical Formulary or Aqrābādhīn of Al-Kindī* (Madison, Wisc., 1966); Nicolas Lemery, *Dictionnaire Universel des Drogues Simples*, ed. nouvelle (Paris, 1759); J. Worth Estes and LaVerne Kuhnke, "French Observations of Disease and Drug Use in Late Eighteenth-Century Cairo," *Journal of the History of Medicine and Allied Sciences 39* (1984): 121–152; T. E. Wallis, *Textbook of Pharmacognosy*, 4th ed. (London, 1960); Maurice Vejux Tyrode, *Pharmacology: the Action and Uses of Drugs* (Philadelphia, 1908); Solomon Solis-Cohen and Thomas Stotesbury Githens, *Pharmacotherapeutics* (New York, 1928); Walter H. Lewis and Memory P. P. Elvin-Lewis, *Medical Botany* (New York, 1977).

Ida Hay at the Arnold Arboretum, Boston, provided important assistance in ascertaining the most recent scientific names for many plant species. Boulos' book provides a great deal of information about modern Egyptians' uses of many ancient botanical drug ingredients. Few of the materials listed in this glossary appear in modern pharmacology texts, and none (save opium derivatives) is exploited regularly in modern American therapeutics.

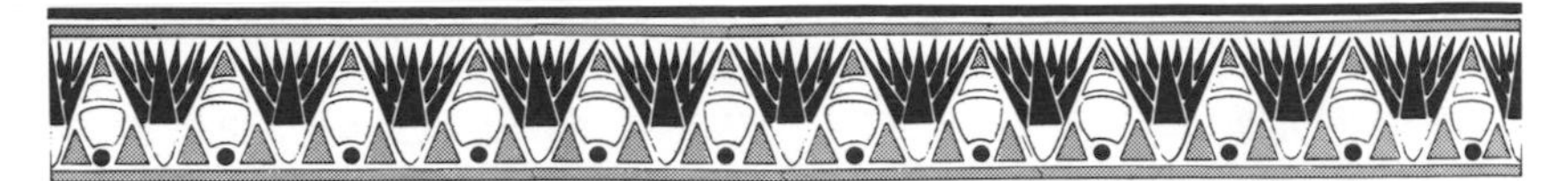

GLOSSARY OF DRUG SUBSTANCES

Abies spp.: see TEREBINTH.

ABSINTHE: bitter extract of wormwood, *Artemisia absinthum*.* 1.54 percent. For respiratory and, chiefly, intestinal disorders. [Used as a potent nerve stimulant in the past.]

ACACIA: leaves or the gum resin of *Acacia nilotica*, or perhaps *A. seyal*.* 6.06 percent. Nonselective, but usually applied topically for sore limbs or superficial skin conditions (especially "swollen glands"). Also see GALL NUTS, GUM AMMONIAC, and GUM, WHITE. [Emulsifier.]

Acacia spp.: see ACACIA.

ALABASTER powder: calcite, a crystalline form of calcium carbonate, $CaCO_3$ (not GYPSUM, q.v., called alabaster elsewhere). 0.59 percent. For skin conditions.

ALKANET: henna, red dye made from the leaves and shoots of the North African species *Lawsonia inermis* or *L. alba**. (This identification is sometimes erroneously confused with *Anchusa tinctoria*, a European species more recently—and confusingly—renamed *Alkanna tinctoria*, which contains an orange dye in its roots.) 0.24 percent. To treat *wḫdw* in the gut.

Allium cepa: see ONION.

Allium kurrat: see LEEK.

Allium porrum: see LEEK.

ALOE: extract of *Aloe* spp.* 1.90 percent. To treat eye diseases. [Laxative, and astringent.]

Aloe sp.: see ALOE.

ALUM: aluminum potassium sulfate, $AlK(SO_4)_2 \cdot 12H_2O$. 0.24 percent. [Externally, an astringent; internally, in low doses an antidiarrheal, and in high doses an emetic.]

Aluminum salts: see ALUM, FELDSPAR, kaolin.

AMMI: an aromatic plant, *Ammi majus* or *A. visnaga* (but possibly same as CUMIN, q.v.). It has been reported that the Egyptians used ammi to treat vitiligo, in which the skin loses its pigmentation in blotchy areas, because people who have eaten the plant are hypersensitive to sunburn (due to the light-activated psoralens contained in ammi); see Richard L. Edelson, "Light-Activated Drugs," *Scientific American 259* (no. 2, August 1988), 68–75. 3.09 percent. Used nonselectively.

Ammi spp.: see AMMI.

ANIMAL BODY PARTS, excluding FAT, GREASE, DUNG, URINE, MILK, AND EGGS. 16.3 percent.

Anethum graveolens: see DILL.

ANISE: seeds of *Pimpinella anisum**. 1.90 percent. Used nonselectively. (Formerly used as a Carminative, q.v.).

ANTELOPE Grease. 0.12 percent. For an anal disorder. Also see GAZELLE, GOAT, IBEX, SHEEP.

Antimony salts: see STIBIUM.

Apium graveolens dulce: see CELERY.

Arsenic salts: see ORPIMENT.

Artemisia absinthum: see ABSINTHE.

ASS Head, Ears, Teeth, Leg Bones, Jaw Marrow, Skin, Grease, Heart, Liver, Testes, Dung, and Milk. 2.73 percent, the third most frequently used animal source of drug materials. Nonselective.

Assafoetida: see SAGAPEN and SILPHIUM.

BALANITES (or BALANOS) OIL: aromatic extract of the kernels of the hegelig thorn tree, *Balanites aegyptica*. 4.16 percent. Used nonselectively.

Balanites aegyptica: see BALANITES OIL.

Balm of Gilead: Same as BALM OF MECCA.

BALM (or BALSAM) OF MECCA: resin of *Commiphora opobalsamum**. 1.66 percent. For eye diseases.

Balsamodendron spp.: see MYRRH.

BARLEY: *Hordeum vulgare* (or, less likely, *H. distichum*) as dry grain or as paste. 3.68 percent. Chiefly for skin conditions.

BAT Blood. 0.12 percent For an eye disorder.

BAYBERRRY (?): probably laurel, or sweet-bay, *Laurus nobilis**. 0.24 percent. Nonselective.

BEANS: exact species unknown; possibilities include "Egyptian bean," the seed of the pink lotus (*Nelumbium speciosum*), the broad bean (*Vicia faba*), or, least likely, the cowpea (*Vigna unguiculata*), q.v.; usually powdered, sometimes mashed. 2.73 percent. Chiefly for skin and musculo-skeletal conditions.

BEER: made from BARLEY, emmer WHEAT, or DATES. 14.49 percent (about same as in Hearst Papyrus). Its alcohol content ranged from 6.2 to 8.1 percent. Although beer is intoxicating and diuretic, it is not clear whether it was included in so many medications for those reasons, or because it was a convenient diluent. Included chiefly in remedies for gut disorders (including worms and diarrhea), but also urinary and musculo-skeletal diseases; never used in remedies for superficial skin wounds. (For brewing techniques, see Lucas, 10–16.)

Beeswax: see WAX.

Beetles: not further identifiable, but possibly powdered "Spanish fly," *Lytta* (formerly *Cantharis*) *vesicatoria*, or perhaps *Mylabris dicinata, M. tripartita*, or *Meloe variegatus*. [Skin vesicant later used as a blistering agent; contains a potent heart toxin called cantharidin.]

Ben Oil: see MORINGA.
BENZOIN: see STYRAX.
Bile: see GALL.
Bindweed: *Convolvulus hystrix*, according to Dawson. Used in treatments for the anus in Chester Beatty VI Papyrus.
BIRDS: unknown species. Brains (for an eye disease), and Heart (for intestinal worms). 0.24 percent. Also see OSTRICH, PELICAN, PIGEON, RAVEN, SWALLOW.
BITUMEN: naturally occurring (but not in Egypt) mixtures of hydrocarbons and other substances, such as wood tar and asphalt. 0.12 percent. For respiratory difficulty.
BLOOD, of OX, BAT, GOOSE, RAVEN, PIGEON, FROG, LIZARD, and FLIES. 1.66 percent. For disorders of skin and eyes.
Bolti fish: see LATES NILOTICA.
BONES: Leg of ASS, DOG, HIPPOPOTAMUS; RAVEN; FISH; CUTTLEFISH; and unknown species. 0.95 percent. For disease of organs of head. Also see MARROW and SKULL.
Boswellia spp.: see FRANKINCENSE.
BRAINS, of OX, PIG, SILURUS FISH. 1.07 percent. Nonselective. Also see HEAD, SKULL.
BRAN: seed husks of unspecified grains. 1.90 percent. Used chiefly for skin diseases.
Brassica nigra: see MUSTARD.
BREAD AND CAKES. 1.54 percent. Used chiefly in gut disorders.
BRICK [dust]. 0.36 percent.
Broad bean: see BEANS.
Bryonia spp.: see BRYONY.
BRYONY, WHITE: berries of *Bryonia dioica** or *B. cretica*. 2.26 percent. Nonselective; also in two remedies for the anus in Chester Beatty VI Papyrus.
Cadmium salts: see SORY.
CALAMINE (?): usually zinc oxides with iron oxides added, but sometimes zinc silicates. 0.59 percent. Used in ointments. [Mild astringent and antiseptic.]
Calamus draco: see DRAGON'S BLOOD.
Calcium salts: see ALABASTER, GYPSUM, LIMESTONE, Memphis stone.
CALOTROPIS: giant milkweed, *Calotropis procera**. 3.68 percent. Used to stimulate the *metu*. Contains an emetic substance and a potent heart stimulant called calotropin—but this does not mean that the drug was used to stimulate the heart in ancient Egypt. Used nonselectively, but mostly for diseases of the urinary tract and limbs. Because the calotropis fruit resembles testicles, it has been suggested that it was meant by the word Ebbell translated as CELERY because the juice within the stalks of *Apium graveolens dulce* has been likened to semen; see Francois Daumas, "Note sur la Plante *Matjet*," *Bulletin de l'Institut Français d'Archéologie Orientale* 56 (1957): 59–66.
Calotropis procera: see CALOTROPIS.
Camphor*: probably CINNAMON*, q.v.

Cannabis sativa: see Marijuana.
Cantharis vesicatoria: see Beetles.
Carduus sp.: see White Thistle.
Carminatives: drugs that expel gas from the stomach or intestines. They illustrate the confusing lack of specificity that can be ascribed to drug usage even into relatively modern times, when they were used in a wide variety of unrelated clinical circumstances such as: intestinal and uterine cramps; abdominal distention; laxative overdoses; worms, rheumatism, asthma, and hysteria; to stimulate nasal secretions; to stimulate healing of chronic skin diseases; as antiseptics and anesthetics; and as diuretics and counterirritants (similar to agents, such as tincture of powdered *Lytta vesicatoria* beetles, q.v., that irritate the skin in order to relieve a more deeply seated inflammatory process by permitting its escape from the body or by antagonizing it). Despite this profusion of clinical indications for their usage, the carminatives were thought to exert all their purported manifold effects via a common action on the gastrointestinal tract (although I can find no data that support the notion that any carminatives truly affected gastrointestinal action). Thus, even if a carminative *did* appear to deflate a bloated intestine or prevent belching, it is improbable that those actions (unlikely as they are) could have provided specific relief for, say, the infectious diseases of the skin or the "prolapsed uterus" which originally brought the patient to the physician in either ancient Egypt or nineteenth-century America.
CAROB: beans of the evergreen tree *Ceratonia siliqua*, although Ebbell translated the Egyptian word as "MANNA" (q.v.). 3.68 percent. Used chiefly for disorders of gut and urinary tract. Is a remedy for all ailments of the anus in the Chester Beatty VI Papyrus, although the translation is not certain (also see *DJARET*). [Formerly used as a laxative, but efficacy doubtful.]
CASSIA: bark or beans of *Cassia fistula**, or perhaps *Cinnamomum cassia*. [Laxative]. Also see MALABATHRON and CINNAMON.
Cassia acutifolia: see SENNA.
Cassia angustifolia: see SENNA.
Cassia fistula: see CASSIA.
CASTOREUM (?): a foul-smelling watery material found in the preputial glands of the beaver, *Castor* spp., but beavers are not known to have lived in Egypt at any time; if Ebbell's translation is correct, the Egyptians must have imported the material from Mesopotamia. 0.12 percent. Used to treat women's diseases.
Castor Oil: see RICINUS.
CAT Hair, Skin, Fat, Uterus, and, most often, Dung. 1.43 percent. Used to treat disease in analogous organs in human patients.
Cattle: see OX.
Cedar: oil or resin from *Cedrus* or related genera (??).
Cedrus: see CEDAR.
CELERY: *Apium graveolens dulce*. However, the correct translation of the Egyptian word is probably CALOTROPIS (q.v.).

Ceratonia siliqua: see CAROB.

CHAFF: 0.12 percent.

CHARCOAL. 0.12 percent. For skin diseases. [An adsorbent].

CHASTE TREE: *Vitex agnus-castus*. 1.78 percent. Used for skin, joint, and intestinal symptoms.

Cinnabar: see DRAGON'S BLOOD.

CINNAMON: probably not the true cinnamon spice, from *Cinnamomum zeylanicum**, which is not native to Egypt (it was imported much later), but *C. cassia* or even *C. camphora**. (For more on this confusion, see Riddle, 98–104.) Also see: MALABATHRON. 1.54 percent. Chiefly for disorders of the skin and limbs. [Mild antiseptic properties; can stimulate respiration in mild circulatory collapse.]

Cinnamomum spp.: see CINNAMON and MALABATHRON.

Cirsium sp.: see White Thistle.

Cistus spp.: see LADANUM.

Citrullus colocynthis: see COLOCYNTH.

Citrullus vulgaris: see WATERMELON.

Citrus aurantifolia: see Lime.

Claviceps purpurea: see ERGOT.

CLAY. 0.48 percent. Perhaps FELDSPAR, or kaolin, q.v. Used for sore limbs and eyes.

CLOVER, SWEET: *Melilotus indica* (Dawson's *M. officinalis* cannot be correct). 1.42 percent. Nonselective.

Cnicus: see White Thistle.

COLOCYNTH: fruit of *Citrullus colocynthis**. 5.34 percent. Used primarily for gut and anal disorders, including worms. [Strong laxative.]

Commiphora abyssinica: see MYRRH.

Commiphora kataf: see Kafal.

Commiphora opobalsamum: see BALM OF MECCA.

Commiphora pedunculata: see FRANKINCENSE.

Convolvulus hystrix: see Bindweed.

COPPER FLAKES: refuse from hammering the metal. 1.19 percent. For disorders of limbs associated with *wḥdw* and for female organs (never for gut). Perhaps acted like MALACHITE, q.v., but doubtful.

Copper Salts: for the prototype see MALACHITE, but others were probably used as well. [Externally, astringent and antiseptic; internally, emetic.]

Cordia myxa: see SEBESTEN.

CORIANDER: seeds of *Coriandrum sativum*. 1.90 percent. For disorders of gut, urination, and *metu* of limbs. [Formerly used as a Carminative, q.v.]

Coriandrum sativum: see CORIANDER.

COSTUS (?): even if Ebbell's translation is correct, he did not specify whether he meant *Costus spicatus*, whose sap is reported to be mildly diuretic, or *Saussurea lappa*, whose root has been used for asthma (although with what success is unreported). 0.59 percent. Nonselective.

Costus spicatus: see COSTUS.

COW: see MILK of COW, and OX.

Cowpea: *Vigna unguiculata* var. *unguiculata* (formerly, *V. sinensis*). In Papyrus Chester Beatty VI, for anal disorders. Also see BEANS.

CREAM: See MILK.

CROCODILE Dung. 0.83 percent. Nonselective, and in a pessary to prevent conception.

Crocus sativus: see SAFFRON.

Croton spp.: see DRAGON'S BLOOD.

CUCUMBER: perhaps *Ecballium elaterium* (sometimes called squirting cucumber), a dangerously laxative and emetic gourd, but only the leaves were recommended by the author of the Ebers papyrus, to treat the *metu*. Although it was not introduced into Egypt until the New Kingdom, today's common edible cucumber (*Cucumis sativus* or *C. chate*) may have been meant by the Ebers author. 0.48 percent. Nonselective.

Cucumis melo: see Melon.

Cucumis sativus: see CUCUMBER.

CUMIN: aromatic seeds of *Cuminum cyminum*. 4.63 percent. Used nonselectively, but not for eye conditions. [Formerly used as a Carminative, q.v.]

Cuminum cyminum: see CUMIN.

CUTTLEFISH (squidlike cephalopods of genus *Sepia*) "bone." 1.19 percent. Nonselective.

Cyperus esculentus sativa: see RUSH-NUT.

Cyperus papyrus: see PAPYRUS.

DATES: fruit of date palm, *Phoenix dactylifera*. 6.89 percent. Used nonselectively, predominantly for gut disorders, but not for superficial skin wounds. Also see BEER.

DATE WINE: made from DATES steeped in water. 2.73 percent. Nonselective, but most often for superficial skin conditions.

DILL: aromatic seeds or leaves of *Anethum graveolens*. 0.24 percent. [Formerly used as a Carminative, q.v.]

Diospyros ebenum: See EBONY.

DJARET: a gourd or fruit that has not yet been positively identified. 14.61 percent, the greatest frequency of occurrence in the Ebers prescriptions (and in the Hearst Papyrus, 12.69 percent) of any single drug ingredient, save honey, that was presumed to be an active principle. All parts of the plant were used nonselectively for all conditions except magically induced disease. CAROB, COLOCYNTH, and Opium have been suggested, but all seem unlikely (for references, see n. 17, Chapter Five).

DOG Leg Bones and Dung. 0.48 percent. For disorders of skin and limbs.

Dorema ammoniacum: see GUM AMMONIAC.

Dracaena sp.: see DRAGON'S BLOOD.

DRAGON'S BLOOD: red pigments from *Calamus draco*, an East Indian palmtree, *Croton* spp., or *Dracaena* spp. However, none of these was found in ancient Egypt; it is more likely to have been Cinnabar, red mercuric sulfide (HgS). 0.71 percent. Nonselective. (For its use in Western medicine see Torald

Sollman, "A Sketch of the History of 'Dragon's Blood,'" *Journal of the American Pharmaceutical Association* 9 [1920]: 141–144.)

DUNG, chiefly of CAT and CROCODILE, then ASS and MAN, but also of PIG, DOG, SHEEP, GAZELLE, PELICAN, and FLIES. 5.23 percent. Nonselective; applied only topically.

EAR, of ASS. 0.12 percent. For an ear disorder.

EBONY flakes (??): perhaps bark or shavings of *Diospyros ebenum*; the English word derives from the Egyptian *hebni*. 0.36 percent. For eye disease.

Ecballium elaterium: see CUCUMBER.

EGGS, chiefly of OSTRICH, but also GOOSE (yolk only) and RAVEN. 1.54 percent. Nonselective, but chiefly for skin and hair conditions. Egyptian bean: see BEANS.

Emmer: See WHEAT.

Ergot: the *Claviceps purpurea* fungus that infests rye, *Secale cereale*. Its medical use in ancient Egypt is doubtful; it is not mentioned in the Ebers Papyrus at any rate, but Leake postulates that it is mentioned in the Hearst Papyrus. [Stimulates uterine contractions, and constricts small arteries.]

EYES, of PIG. 0.12 percent. For eye disease.

FAIENCE: glazed pottery fragments. 0.24 percent.

FAT, chiefly of GOOSE, but also of OX, CAT, HIPPOPOTAMUS, MOUSE, OSTRICH, and SNAKE. 4.75 percent, and in about 1 to 5 percent of Hearst prescriptions. Nonselective, and perhaps used as an inactive vehicle for presumed active drug ingredients, especially (but not exclusively) those prepared for topical application. Also see GREASE.

FELDSPAR: aluminum silicates with certain impurities, but probably same as kaolin*, q.v. Also see CLAY. [An adsorbent, kaolin is still used in remedies for diarrhea.]

Fennel: seeds or stalks of *Foeniculum vulgare*. [Formerly used as a Carminative, q.v.]

Ferula spp.: see SAGAPEN and SILPHIUM.

Ficus carica: see FIGS.

Ficus sycomorus: see SYCOMORE.

FIGS: fruit of *Ficus carica* (but also see SYCOMORE). 5.23 percent. Used nonselectively to correct disordered *metu* associated with disease of skin, gut, and urinary tract. [Mild laxative].

FISH Brains, Head, and Bones, of many species (probably including *Tilapia nilotica, Synodontis schall*, and *Mugil cephalus*. 0.48 percent. For disorders of skin, head, and eyes. Also see LATES NILOTICA, SILURUS FISH, and TADPOLES.

FLAX (?): made from fibers of *Linum usitatissimum* (and perhaps other species). 0.71 percent. Nonselective.

FLAX-SEED. 1.31 percent. Nonselective.

FLESH: see MEAT.

FLINT: fragments of a hard, fine-grained quartz also flaked to make a sharp cutting edge. 0.71 percent. Used in topical remedies applied to head.

FLIES: Blood (seems unlikely to be an accurate literal translation), Whole Fly, but chiefly Dung, are specified. 1.66 percent. Used externally nonselectively, although most often for skin disease and wounds.

Foeniculum vulgare: see Fennel.

FRANKINCENSE: fragrant gum-resin from *Boswellia carteri** and other species, e.g., *B. sacra* or *Commiphora pedunculata*. 14.13 percent. Used nonselectively, often to treat disordered *metu* (perhaps its fragrance was thought to counter the stench of *wḫdw*).

Fraxinus ornus: see MANNA.

FRIT: artificially manufactured crystals, like those of glass or faience, made with calcium-copper silicate, calcite, alkalies such as natron, and copper or iron pigments. 0.36 percent. For skin disease and wounds.

FROG Blood. 0.12 percent. For skin disease. Also see TADPOLE.

GALENA: lead sulfide, PbS, the principal ore of lead. 8.19 percent, if this is the correct translation of the word Ebbell translated as STIBIUM (q.v.).

GALL, chiefly of OX, but also of GOAT, TORTOISE, an unidentified bird, and HUMANS. 1.54 percent. Nonselective, but chiefly for eye and superficial skin conditions.

GALL NUTS: external plant swellings caused by insects, microorganisms, or injury, from several kinds of trees, including ACACIA and TAMARIX. 0.59 percent. Applied topically but nonselectively. [Contain astringent or styptic tannins that are still sometimes applied to burns.]

GAZELLE Horn, Dung. 0.36 percent. Chiefly for skin disease.

Glass: see FRIT.

GOAT Meat, Gall. 0.36 percent. For skin conditions.

GOOSE FAT and GREASE, as well as Blood and Egg Yolks. 5.24 percent, the second most frequently used animal drug ingredient. The FAT and GREASE were probably used as vehicles for drugs that were presumed to be active, especially those that were to be applied to the skin.

Gourd: probably COLOCYNTH (q.v.), possibly CUCUMBER (q.v.).

GRANITE flakes. 0.36 percent. For skin and eye disorders.

GRAPES: fruit of *Vitis vinifera* (which also produced RAISINS and WINE). 2.26 percent. Used nonselectively, especially to treat disorders of *metu* to various organs.

GREASE, chiefly of OX, but also of GOOSE, ASS, PIG, ANTELOPE, IBEX. 9.50 percent. Nonselective, and perhaps used as an inactive vehicle for presumed active drug ingredients, especially (but not exclusively) those prepared for topical application. Also see: FAT.

GRUB WORMS, species unknown, apparently whole: 0.12 percent. For skin disease.

Gum: probably most often from ACACIA (q.v.).

GUM AMMONIAC (?), from *Dorema ammoniacum**, but more likely to have been gum of ACACIA, q.v. 0.83 percent. Nonselective. [Formerly used as an expectorant, antispasmodic, laxative, diuretic, and tonic, all probably in vain.]

Gum Arabic: see ACACIA.

GUM, WHITE, possibly from ACACIA, q.v. 5.23 percent. Used nonselectively for external ailments, especially of the associated *metu*; perhaps used only as a binding agent or vehicle.

GYPSUM: calcium sulfate, $CaSO_4 \cdot 2H_2O$. 0.83 percent. Used to treat skin and limb wounds. [A major ingredient of, e.g., plaster-of-Paris.]

HAIR, of CAT. 0.12 percent. For skin injury.

HEAD, whole, of ASS (for disorder in the belly), MOUSE (for sore limbs) and a FISH (for a head ailment), although these seem unlikely to have been meant to be taken literally. 0.36 percent. Also see BRAINS, EARS, EYES, HORN, SKULL and TEETH.

HEART, of ASS (for sore limbs) and unknown bird species (for worms). 0.24 percent.

HEDGEHOG prickles. 0.24 percent. For skin disorders. In other texts, hedgehog fat is said to cure baldness. The animal also had other magical protective properties.

Hegelig: see BALANITES.

Hematite: see OCHRE, RED.

Henbane: see HYOSCYAMUS.

Henna: see ALKANET.

HIPPOTAMUS Leg Bones, Skin, but chiefly Fat. 0.95 percent. Usually for skin ointments, but also for gut disorders.

HONEY, probably from domestic hives. 30.29 percent; about 40 percent among Hearst prescriptions. The most frequently used of all drug ingredients, it was applied nonselectively to disorders of all organ systems. The *swnw* probably thought it was an active ingredient, not merely a vehicle or diluent for other drug materials. One major use was as a wound dressing. (For Egyptian bee-keeping, see Lucas, *Ancient Egyptian Materials*, 25–26, and Eva Crane, *The Archaeology of Beekeeping* (Ithaca, N.Y., 1983), 35–39.) [Antiseptic properties; see Chapter Three.] Also see WAX.

Hordeum spp.: see BARLEY.

HORN, of GAZELLE, ground. 0.12 percent. For skin disease.

HUMAN Gall (which seems unlikely to be an accurate literal translation), Dung, Urine of Males, and MILK OF A WOMAN WHO HAS DELIVERED A MALE CHILD (q.v.). 2.49 percent, most often as the latter product.

HYOSCYAMUS: probably Egyptian henbane, *Hyoscyamus muticus*, but perhaps *H. albus** or *H. niger*. 1.66 percent. Used for ailments of the limbs and gut. This or a closely related species was probably the major poisonous plant in ancient Egypt; A. Lucas, "Poison in Ancient Egypt," *Journal of Egyptian Archaeology 24* (1938): 198–199. [Its principal alkaloid, scopolamine, has atropine-like effects; it produces drowsiness, euphoria, and dreamless sleep, and slows both the pulse and gut activity]. Also see discussion of Mandrake in Chapter Five.

Hyoscyamus spp.: see HYOSCYAMUS.

IBEX Grease. 1.07 percent. Nonselective.

INDIGO: blue dye from *Indigofera* spp., perhaps *I. argentea*. 0.24 percent. Used in gut disorders.

Indigofera spp.: see INDIGO.

INK-POWDER: finely divided carbon particles, generally from soot, for making black ink (also see SOOT and OCHRE, RED). 2.38 percent. Used nonselectively, but seldom for diseases of internal organs.

IRON salts: see MAGNETITE, OCHRE, RED, and OCHRE, YELLOW.

Ished tree: see SEBESTEN.

IVORY, source not specified. 0.12 percent. For skin disease.

Jujubes: see ZIZYPHUS.

Juncus spp.: see RUSH-NUT.

JUNIPER: probably berries or other plant parts of *Juniperus phoenicea*, but perhaps *J. communis*, *J. drupacea*, or *J. oxycedrus*. 6.18 percent. Used nonselectively but not for eye diseases or skin wounds. [Formerly used as an astringent and to promote menstrual flow.]

Juniperus spp.: see JUNIPER.

Kafal: aromatic gum from *Commiphora kataf**.

Kaolin*: a fine soft clay of pure $Al_2O_3 \cdot SiO_2 \cdot 2H_2O$. Also see FELDSPAR. [Still used, for its absorbent properties, as an antidiarrheal agent.]

Lactuca spp.: see Lettuce.

LADANUM: aromatic resin from *Cistus ladanifer* and perhaps other species, e.g., *C. creticus**. 1.78 percent. Used chiefly for disorders of skin and hair.

LAPIS LAZULI: powdered dark blue stone containing sodium and aluminum silicates, and sodium sulfide, laced with white calcite (calcium carbonate, $CaCO_3$) and gold flecks of iron pyrite ("fool's gold," FeS_2). Its closest source was modern Afghanistan. 0.36 percent. For eye disorders.

Larix spp.: larch; see TEREBINTH.

LATES NILOTICA: *Tilapia nilotica*, a Nile catfish also known as the bolti. It was a symbol of fecundity because its young are hatched in the adult's mouth. 0.12 percent. For women's disorders.

Laurus nobilis: see BAYBERRY.

Lawsonia spp.: see ALKANET.

Lead salts: see GALENA and MINIUM.

LEATHER, BURNT: 0.12 percent. For superficial wounds.

LEEK: *Allium kurrat* or perhaps *A. porrum* (or perhaps ONION, *Allium cepa*, q.v.) 0.24 percent. For superficial wounds.

Lettuce: probably *Lactuca virosa*, which is not our garden lettuce (*L. sativa*, which is said to have been used as a food in Egypt). Its milky juice enhanced its association with the priapic Egyptian fertility god Min. [*L. virosa* was used occasionally in later Western medicine as a narcotic and diuretic, but in vain.]

Lime: *Citrus aurantifolia*, but this translation is impossible to verify; it is uncertain that the tree grew in ancient Egypt, and there is little if any convincing evidence that scurvy was a problem there, despite Ebbell's unlikely interpretation of the term "blood-eating" as scurvy. Limes do, of course, contain vitamin C, the antiscorbutic vitamin, but that does not necessarily mean that the Egyptians used limes to treat what we now recognize as scurvy.

LIMESTONE: powdered calcium carbonate, $CaCO_3$. Nonselective. 0.36 percent. [Externally, an astringent; internally, an antidiarrheal.]

Linum spp.: see FLAX.

Liquidambar orientalis: see STYRAX.

LIVER, of OX, ASS, SWALLOW. 0.48 percent. Nonselective. Also see GALL. Beef liver is a major source of vitamin A, a deficiency of which results in night blindness, for which an Ebers prescription recommends cooked liver. The first prescription of the Kahun Papyrus recommends raw ass liver for a woman with poor vision attributable to uterine disease.

LIZARD Blood, and Dung. 0.48 percent. For eye diseases.

LOTUS, or Water Lily, *Nymphaea* spp.* 0.59 percent. Nonselective. A recent hypothesis is that lotus was used for its potential but unverified narcotic properties (W. Benson Harer, Jr., "Pharmacological and Biological Properties of the Egyptian Lotus," *Journal of the American Research Center in Egypt 22* [1985]: 49–54). Also see BEANS, PONDWEED, and POTAMOGETON.

LYE (?): potassium hydroxide, KOH. 0.12 percent. For *metu* of gut.

Lytta vesicatoria: see Beetles.

MAGNETITE: black iron oxide, Fe_3O_4. 0.24 percent. For superficial disorders of head. Also see OCHRE, RED and OCHRE, YELLOW.

MALABATHRON: leaves of a *Cinnamomum* species, perhaps *C. zeylanicum* or *C. tamala*, but possibly of CASSIA (q.v.) as well. 0.12 percent. For female disorders.

MALACHITE: a bright green copper ore, characteristically layered in cross-section, composed chiefly of cupric carbonate, $CuCo_3 \cdot Cu(OH)_2 \cdot H_2O$; probably the "powdered green pigment" of the Smith Papyrus. 4.63 percent. Used nonselectively, but especially for eye disease and as a wound dressing; never for disorders of the chest or applied directly to the female organs. [Antiseptic properties; see Chapter Three.]

MAN: see HUMAN.

MANNA: resin of *Fraxinus ornus*, which was probably not used in ancient Egypt; see CAROB.

Marijuana: *Cannabis sativa** cannot be positively identified in the Ebers or Hearst papyri, although it may be the *šmšmt* which is in one Ebers prescription for sore limbs and another for female disorders, according to Dawson. Marijuana may also be an ingredient of an anal remedy in the Chester Beatty VI Papyrus. It grew easily and widely in Egypt, and was used there for its euphoric effect by the late eighteenth century A.D., but neither the Greeks nor Romans used it as an intoxicant (Theodore F. Brunner, "Marijuana in Ancient Greece and Rome? The Literary Evidence," *Bulletin of the History of Medicine 47* [1973]: 344–355).

MARROW of OX leg and ASS jaw. 0.95 percent. Nonselective, but used most often for eye disease. Also see: BONE.

MEAT, fresh, or decayed in one instance, chiefly of OX, but also of GOAT, SHEEP, and SILURUS FISH. 2.26 percent. Nonselective, but used most often for sore limbs; also applied to wounds.

MECCA BALSAM: see BALM OF MECCA.

Melilotus spp.: see CLOVER, SWEET.

Meloe variegatus: see Beetles.

Melon: *Cucumis melo*, whose many varieties include the wintermelon, muskmelon, and cantaloupe. In Papyrus Chester Beatty VI, for a hot anus.

Memphis Stone: a form of calcium carbonate known not from Egyptian papyri but from Dioscorides and Pliny; said to have produced analgesia.

Mentha: see Mint.

Mercury salts: see DRAGON'S BLOOD (for Cinnabar).

MILK of ASS. 0.48 percent. For gut and skin afflictions.

MILK of COW. 3.80 percent (about same among the Hearst recipes); cream was specified in another 0.36 percent of Ebers recipes. Nonselective (but not used in urinary tract remedies).

MILK OF A WOMAN WHO HAS DELIVERED A MALE CHILD. 1.66 percent. Used nonselectively for superficial disorders, not for diseases of internal organs.

MILLIPEDES, sp. unknown, probably whole or crushed. 0.12 percent. For skin disease.

MILLSTONE SCRAPINGS: 0.36 percent. For superficial injuries.

Mimusops Schimperi: see SEBESTEN.

MINIUM: red lead, lead oxide, Pb_3O_4. However, this translation is probably not accurate. Dawson proposed that yellow iron oxide (see OCHRE, YELLOW) was really meant, and Lucas argues that minium did not appear in Egypt before the Roman conquest. Metallic lead itself did not come into common use, for items such as fish net sinkers and statuettes, before the New Kingdom (H.A. Waldron, "Lead Poisoning in the Ancient World," *Medical History 17* [1973]: 391–399). 0.71 percent. Used chiefly for sore limbs. [Formerly used in wound dressings and plasters.] Also see GALENA.

Mint: probably *Mentha longifolia*, but possibly *M. pulegium, M. spicata*, or another species. [Formerly used as a Carminative, q.v., and to relieve the stomach pains of ulcer patients.]

MORINGA: sweet odorless oil from the ben-nut (sometimes called horse radish tree), *Moringa aptera* or *M. pterygosperma*.* Associated with Osiris, it was prized because it does not easily become rancid. 0.12 percent. For worms.

Moringa spp.: see MORINGA.

MOUSE Head (for an ear disease) and Fat (for a musculo-skeletal disorder). 0.24 percent. (Also see Chapter Five).

MUSSELS, Freshwater: a proposed translation of *wḏ'jt*. 1.31 percent. Used nonselectively.

MUSTARD: perhaps *Brassica* or *Sinapis nigra*, or *S. alba*. 0.83 percent. For disorders of limbs and gut. (Externally, rubefacient; internally, in large doses, emetic.)

Mylabris spp.: see Beetles.

MYRRH: fragrant gum-resin probably from *Commiphora abyssinica**, but possibly from *Balsamodendron* species. 5.23 percent. Nonselective, but used chiefly for skin, limb, and gut afflictions (not those of the chest). [Said to be astringent and antiseptic, but see Chapter Three.]

MYRTLE (?): probably *Myrtus communis*, an evergreen shrub, but any one of many other plants, such as *Piper* spp.*, may have been meant. 2.49 percent. An astringent used nonselectively, but not for eyes.

Myrtus communis: see MYRTLE.

NAPHTHA (?): this translation is unlikely, since petroleum products were unknown in ancient Egypt; perhaps the Ebers Papyrus author meant a bright blue "naphtha salt" found in Persia which gives off an odor of naphtha. 0.12 percent. For eyes.

NATRON and RED NATRON, naturally occurring mixtures of sodium carbonate, Na_2CO_3 ("washing soda") and sodium bicarbonate, $NaHCO_3$ ("baking soda"), with impurities including high proportions of SALT (NaCl), q.v., and sodium sulfate ($NaSO_4$). The ancient Egyptian word for natron, *ntry*, is said to have given rise to the modern word niter, which is potassium nitrate (KNO_3), or saltpeter. Red natron was specified only one-third as frequently as natron. 6.29 percent (and in 7.31 percent of Hearst prescriptions). Used externally, sometimes to treat disordered *metu*, for skin and limb ailments, and for a few gut disorders. The carbonate is an external rubefacient, and the bicarbonate can reduce stomach acidity, purposes for which natron may have been recommended by the Ebers papyrus author even though he could not have known about the relationship of peptic ulcer pains to gastric acid. Natron's role in dessicating mummies is discussed in Chapter Two.

Nelumbium speciosum: see BEANS.

Nest, of a bird. Probably used magically.

NORTHERN SALT: see SALT.

Nymphaea spp.: see LOTUS.

OAKUM TAR (?): probably a resin. 0.24 percent. For skin and women's disorders.

OCHRE, RED: red iron oxides, especially Fe_2O_3, hematite. 4.87 percent. Used nonselectively, chiefly for external ailments; also used in red ink. [Externally, an astringent; internally, may cause stomach pain.] Also see: MAGNETITE.

OCHRE, YELLOW: yellowish iron oxides, $FeO(OH) \cdot nH_2O$. 8.19 percent. Used nonselectively for both internal and external ailments, and to correct disordered *metu*. Also see MINIUM.

OIL, ROCK, or MINERAL. 0.24 percent. Perhaps used as an active ingredient, for internal disorders.

OIL, WHITE (or PURE). 14.25 percent; and about twice as frequently among the Hearst prescriptions. Perhaps imported; olives (*Olea europea*) were not introduced into Egypt until Dynasty XVIII. Nonselective; probably used only as a vehicle.

Olibanum: same as FRANKINCENSE.

Olives: see OIL, WHITE.

ONION: *Allium cepa** (or perhaps LEEK or GARLIC, q.v.). 1.31 percent. Nonselective.

Onopordon spp.: see White Thistle.

Opium: Opium (from *Papaver somniferum**) seems not to have been used before the New Kingdom, if then, and at that time it must have been imported. However, *P. somniferum* was being cultivated by Roman times, and that produced at Thebes was then exported all over the known world until modern times; it was the standard against which all others were judged. (See n. 17, Chapter Five, for references.) Also see *DJARET* (which may mean opium) and Poppy Seeds.

ORPIMENT (?): lemon-yellow arsenic trisulfide, As_2S_3, or possibly realgar, which is orange-red arsenic disulfide, As_2S_2. 0.24 percent. Prescribed for upper respiratory symptoms. [Used today in tanning leather.]

OSTRICH Fat, but most often Eggs. 1.07 percent. Chiefly for skin problems, but also for eye disease.

OX Blood, Brains, Leg Marrow, Fat, Flesh (Meat), Liver, Gall, Spleen, and Urine, but chiefly Grease and Milk. 12.29 percent, the most frequently used animal source of drug ingredients. Nonselective.

Palm: see DATES. Other palms were used for food.

PANICLES: loosely branched flower clusters of REED (q.v.) and several other unidentified plants.

Papaver rhoeas: a poppy species that contains far less Opium (q.v.) than *P. somniferum**. It may have been meant by the word *špnn*, recommended in the Smith Papyrus for making a poultice, and in the Ebers Papyrus for a scalp ointment and, mixed with fly's dirt, to quiet a crying child. Also see Poppy Seeds.

*Papaver somniferum**: see Opium and Poppy Seeds.

PAPYRUS strips: from *Cyperus papyrus*. 0.36 percent. Apparently used as bandaging. Also see Chapter Five.

PASTE-WATER (?). 0.12 percent. For women's disorders. See: WHEAT.

Peas: seeds of *Pisum sativum* or *P. arvense*. However, it is possible that the author of the Hearst Papyrus meant another pod-bearing legume, e.g., CASSIA, q.v. Also see: BEANS.

PELICAN Dung. 0.12 percent. For skin disease.

Persea tree: see SEBESTEN.

Phoenix dactylifera: see DATES.

PIG Brains, Eyes, Teeth, Grease, and Dung. 0.83 percent. Nonselective.

PIGEON Blood. 0.12 percent. For skin disease.

PIGNONS: seeds from cones of *Pinus pinea* or other *Pinus* species. 4.63 percent. Nonselective (for all but women's diseases). Also see PINE.

Pimpinella anisum: see ANISE.

PINE TAR. 1.07 percent. Nonselective for external disorders. Also see: TEREBINTH.

PINE, WOOD or SAWDUST: from unidentified species, perhaps *Pinus halepen-*

sis. 1.31 percent. Used for limb, skin, and women's disorders. Also see PIGNONS.

*Pinus** spp.: see PIGNONS, PINE TAR, PINE WOOD, and Terebinth.

Piper spp.: see MYRTLE.

Pistachia spp.: see PISTACIA and Terebinth.

PISTACIA, pistachio: probably *Pistachia atlantica* (but possibly *P. vera**). 0.71 percent. Nonselective. Also see Terebinth.

Pisum spp.: see Peas.

Plum, Egyptian: see SEBESTEN.

POMEGRANATE: roots and fruits of *Punica granatum**. Introduced to Egypt in Dynasty XVIII. 0.24 percent. For intestinal worms. [A mild laxative, still used as a vermifuge in Egypt.]

PONDWEED: species unknown (but also see LOTUS and POTAMOGETON). 0.48 percent. For musculo-skeletal and women's disorders.

Poppy Seeds: from a yet unidentified source. If any poppy species grew in Egypt before the New Kingdom, it was probably *Papaver rhoeas* (q.v.), which may have some slight narcotic effect; the opium poppy, *P. somniferum**, had appeared by the sixteenth century B.C.; see *DJARET* and Opium. [Although the seeds of the opium poppy may sometimes contain trace amounts of morphine and related compounds, the seeds themselves have not been found to possess any related pharmacological activity, although they do contain a hydroscopic oil.]

PORRIDGE (?). 1.66 percent. Nonselective, for *metu* of various organs.

POTAMOGETON: a floating pondweed, *Potamageton* spp. 0.24 percent. For intestinal worms. Also see LOTUS.

Potamageton spp.: see POTAMOGETON.

PUMICE dust. (Although Egypt had no volcanic landscape, pumice could have been brought from eastern Mediterranean sites such as Thera by the New Kingdom.) 0.36 percent. For skin disorders.

Punica granatum: see POMEGRANATE.

RAISINS (?). 2.49 percent. See GRAPES. Used chiefly for disorders of the intestines.

RAM Skin. 0.12 percent. For skin wounds. Also see SHEEP.

RAVEN Blood, Bones, and Eggs. 0.36 percent. For hair and skin conditions.

Realgar: see ORPIMENT.

RED NATRON: see NATRON.

RED OCHRE: see OCHRE, RED.

REED PANICLES. 0.24 percent. For skin and women's disorders.

REED PITH: from any of several tall grass genera. 0.12 percent. For women's disorders.

Reed Stems: may have been sharpened for puncturing and draining abscesses.

Ricinus communis: see RICINUS.

RICINUS seed and oil: castor bean, from *Ricinus communis**. 0.95 percent. For diseases of gut, head, and skin, especially when associated with disordered *metu*. Although castor oil is a well-documented laxative, it was also used externally, for example, as a skin emollient, in ancient Egypt and elsewhere in the ancient world. See Chapter Five for a detailed ancient Egyptian description of its therapeutic effects. For its translations, see: D. Brent Sandy, "Egyptian Terms for Castor," *Chronique d'Égypte* 62 (1987): 49–52.

RUSH-NUT: probably the Nut-Sedge, or Zulu Nut, *Cyperus esculentus*, var. *sativa**, but perhaps the Hard Rush, *Juncus inflexus* (which has been reported to cause toxic symptoms in cattle) or *J. acutus*. 4.16 percent. Nonselective.

Saccharomyces spp.: see YEAST.

SAFFRON: dried stigmas of *Crocus sativus**. 0.36 percent. Probably not grown in Egypt. Nonselective.

SAGAPEN: probably gum from *Ferula persica*, similar to that from assafoetida, *Ferula asa-fetida**, or perhaps Fennell, q.v. 0.95 percent. Chiefly for eye diseases.

Salix safsaf: see WILLOW BUDS.

SALT and NORTHERN SALT: Both are probably sodium chloride, NaCl; the difference between them, if any, is not known, but "northern salt" was specified nine times more often than "salt". 10.33 percent. A red salt harvested from a lake near Memphis, which is in northern Egypt, was mentioned by Pliny (Lucas, *Ancient Egyptian Materials*, 268). Used nonselectively, although seldom on head or eyes. [Externally as an astringent; internally, as a laxative and antidiuretic, in sufficient dose.] Also see NATRON.

SAND. 0.24 percent. Nonselective.

Saussurea lappa: see COSTUS.

Scribe's Pigment: see INK-POWDER and OCHRE, RED.

SEBESTEN: according to Ebbell, the plum-like fruit of *Cordia myxa*, but recent lexicons identify this plant (*ished* in the Ebers Papyrus) as the persea tree, *Mimusops schimperi*, which has no known pharmacological effect, but it did have religious associations for the Egyptians. 4.51 percent. Used nonselectively, but not for disorders of the eyes or for skin injuries. [Laxative.]

Secale cereale: Rye. See ERGOT.

SENNA: leaves of *Cassia angustifolia** or *C. acutifolia**, although CASSIA (q.v.) may have been meant by the Ebers Papyrus author. 1.07 percent. Used chiefly as a laxative, but also for excessive phlegm. [Laxative.]

SESAME: seeds of *Sesamum indicum** or *S. orientale*, but translation not sure. 0.24 percent. Nonselective.

Sesamum spp.: see SESAME.

SHEEP Flesh (for sore limbs), and Dung (for skin wounds). 0.36 percent. Also see RAM.

SHREWMOUSE: see MOUSE.

SILPHIUM (?): probably an extract from *Ferula tingitana*, a North African umbellifer called laser wort or laserpitum, but possibly *F. communis, F. marmarica*, or *F. cyrenaica*. However, Boulos and others identify *Thapsia garganica*, a dangerously potent laxative, as silphium. 2.73 percent. Used for disorders of the gut, limbs, and skin, it was also a symbol of pharaonic vigor. After 100 A.D. siliphium, whatever it was, was replaced by *Ferula asa-fetida* in Roman trade. Both Hippocrates and Roman physicians recommended silphium as a nonselective purgative (see Chalmers L. Gemmill, "Silphium," *Bulletin of the History of Medicine 40* [1966]: 295–313.)

SILURUS FISH: Brains, Skull, and Meat of a Nile catfish, possibly a *Tilapia* sp. 0.59 percent. For skin and joint conditions.

Sinapis spp.: see MUSTARD.

SKINS, of ASS, CAT, HIPPOPOTAMUS, RAM, SNAKE. 0.95 percent. For skin conditions.

SKULL of SILURUS FISH (q.v.). 0.24 percent. For skin wounds.

SNAKE Skin and Fat, of unknown species. 0.48 percent. For skin conditions.

Sodium salts: see NATRON and SALT.

SOOT. 0.24 percent. For sore limbs. (Also see INK-POWDER.)

SORY: a cadmium ore, principally the sulfate, $CdSO_4$. 2.02 percent. Used nonselectively, but primarily to treat diseased *metu* of the gut.

SPELT: a hardy wheat, *Triticum spelta*. 0.12 percent. For women's disorders.

SPLEEN of OX. 0.71 percent. For disorders of limbs and phallus.

STAGHORN: perhaps an antelope's horns. 0.12 percent. For a disease in the head.

STARCH. 0.36 percent. Nonselective.

STIBIUM: an antimony ore, perhaps the pure element or the trisulfide, Sb_2S_3. Inasmuch as antimony ores are not found in Egypt, Lucas argues that this material was much more likely to have been GALENA (q.v.), although he does note that antimony ores are found in areas with which the Egyptians were in contact. 8.19 percent. Used primarily for eye disease, more than any other ingredient in the Ebers Papyrus. [Caustic.]

STORAX: see STYRAX.

STYRAX: benzoin, a resin* collected from *Liquidambar orientalis* or perhaps from *Styrax officinalis*; however, Leake identifies the same Egyptian word in the Hearst Papyrus as "garlic" (*Allium sativum*). 1.19 percent. Nonselective.

Styrax officinalis: see STYRAX.

Sulfur: perhaps pure raw crystalline sulfur. [Externally, irritant and perhaps antiseptic; internally, a mild laxative, by virtue of its biotransformation in the gastrointestinal tract to hydrogen sulfide, H_2S.]

SWALLOW Liver. 0.12 percent. For a female disorder.

SWEET CLOVER: see CLOVER, SWEET.

SYCOMORE: chiefly the sap, but occasionally the fruits or leaves, of *Ficus sycomorus* (sometimes called Egyptian mulberry); sacred to Isis and Hathor. 5.23 percent. Nonselective for *metu* of several organ systems (but not used for eyes or women's disorders). The sap and leaves are still used in Egyptian folk remedies for burns and other skin ailments.

TADPOLE (whole animal). 0.24 percent. For superficial disorders of limbs, but also for earache (Frans Jonckheere, "Prescriptions médicales sur ostraca hiératiques," *Chronique d' Égypte* 29 [1954]: 46–61).

Tamarind: see TAMARIX.

Tamarindus indica: see TAMARIX.
TAMARISK: same as TAMARIX (q.v.).
TAMARIX: any of several small evergreens, e.g., *Tamarix aphylla*, or *T. nilotica*, but the author of the Ebers Papyrus may have meant tamarinds, the large acidic fruit of *Tamarindus indica** which has laxative properties not shared by *Tamarix* species. 1.07 percent. Nonselective.
Tamarix spp.: see TAMARIX.
TEETH, of ASS or PIG. 0.48 percent. Nonselective.
Terebinth: turpentine-like materials from *Pistachia terebinthus* or any of several genera of evergreens such as *Abies, Pinus*, and *Larix*; probably same as TURPENTINE (q.v.) in the Ebers Papyrus.
TESTES, of ASS. 0.12 percent. For diseased limbs.
Thapsia spp.: see SILPHIUM.
Thistle: see WHITE THISTLE.
THYME (?): *Thymus capitatus* or other spp. 1.19 percent. Nonselective.
Thymus spp.: see THYME.
Tilapia nilotica: see LATES NILOTICA.
TORTOISE Gall (for eye disease), but chiefly Shell (nonselective). 0.95 percent.
Triticum spelta: see SPELT.
Triticum dicoccum: see WHEAT.
TURPENTINE. 2.49 percent. Nonselective. Also see Terebinth.
URINE, of HUMAN male, and of OX. 0.36 percent. Nonselective.
UTERUS, of CAT. 0.12 percent. For skin disease.
Vicia faba: see BEANS.
Vigna unguiculata: see BEANS, and Cowpea.
Vitex agnus-castus: see CHASTE TREE.
Vitis vinifera: see GRAPES, RAISINS, and WINE.
WATER: in over 50 percent of both Hearst and Ebers recipes, probably as a vehicle or as a convenient diluent.
Water Lily: see LOTUS.
WATERMELON: *Citrullus vulgaris*. 0.71 percent. Chiefly for gut disorders.
WAX: the only wax known to have been used in ancient Egypt was beeswax. 4.39 percent; and in about 13 percent of Hearst recipes, perhaps as a binding agent, but also as an adhesive for bandages, and as a presumably active ingredient when given internally for gut disorders.
WHEAT: probably emmer, *Triticum dicoccum*, as bran, paste, and kernels. 2.97 percent. Nonselective.
WHITE GUM: see GUM, WHITE.
WHITE OIL: see OIL, WHITE.
White Thistle: the plants we recognize as thistles belong to several genera, including *Carduus, Cirsium, Cnicus*, and *Onopordon*, all in the aster family. [Actual pharmacological activity is doubtful, although *Cnicus japonicus* was once thought to stimulate menstrual flow.]
WILLOW BUDS: from the Egyptian willow, *Salix safsaf*. 0.48 percent. Nonselective.

WINE, both red and white. 5.23 percent, and in about 5 percent of Hearst prescriptions. Probably not used merely, or only, as a vehicle or diluent for other presumably active drug materials because wine appears only in remedies for diseases of the skin, musculo-skeletal system, gut, and female organs, but in no medicine for skin wounds, diseases, the urinary tract, or any part of the head. The association of wine with the benevolence of Osiris may have contributed to its inclusion in at least some medicines. Also see: DATE WINE. (For Egyptian winemaking, see Lucas, 16–24.)

WORMS: see GRUB WORMS.

WORMWOOD: See ABSINTHE.

YEAST: the fungus genus *Saccharomyces*. 1.54 percent. Nonselective.

YELLOW OCHRE: see OCHRE, YELLOW.

Zinc salts: see Calamine.

ZIZYPHUS: probably *Zizphyus spina-Christi* but perhaps *Z. lotus*, or *Z. abyssinica*, from which an alcoholic beverage is made; some species are used for shellacs, and jujube fruits come from others. 1.66 percent. Nonselective.

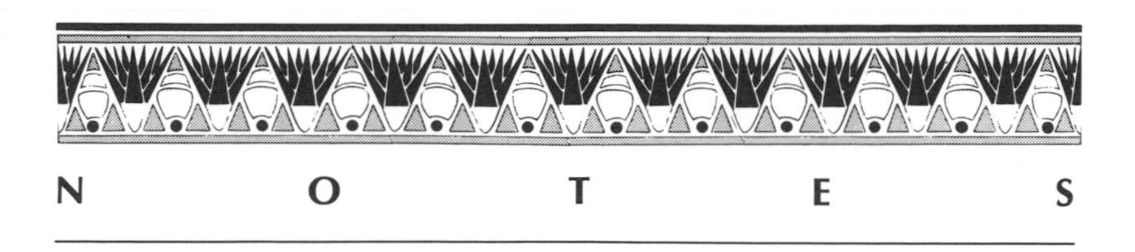

N O T E S

PROLOGUE

1. Sir William Osler, *The Evolution of Modern Medicine* (New Haven, Conn., 1923), 10.
2. Gordon Childe, *What Happened in History* (1942; rev. ed., Harmondsworth, England, 1964), 89–94, 121–132, 159–164, 190–200; Guido Majno, *The Healing Hand: Man and Wound in the Ancient World* (Cambridge, Mass., 1975), 86–89. For an easily available and well-illustrated overview of Imhotep's Egypt, see: Cyril Aldred, *Egypt to the End of the Old Kingdom* (1965; rprt. ed. New York, 1978), and *Egyptian Art* (New York, 1980), especially 11–58. For wheels, see: M. A. Littauer and J. H. Crouwel, "The Earliest Known Three-Dimensional Evidence for Spoked Wheels," *American Journal of Archaeology 90* (1986): 395–398. Throughout this book I have used the dynastic and regnal dates given in John Baines and Jaromír Málek, *Atlas of Ancient Egypt* (New York, 1980), 36–37.
3. Jamieson B. Hurry, *Imhotep: The Vizier and Physician of King Zoser*, 2nd ed. (London, 1928), 4–5; Ange-Pierre Leca, *La Médecine Égyptienne au Temps des Pharaons* (Paris, 1971), 91; Sir Alan Gardiner, *Egypt of the Pharaohs* (London, 1961), 433. Hurry's is the only "biography" of Imhotep; his slimmer 1926 first edition was reprinted (Chicago) in 1978. The surviving documents pertaining to Imhotep have been assembled in Dietrich Wildung, *Egyptian Saints: Deification in Pharaonic Egypt* (New York, 1977), and in his *Imhotep und Amenhotep. Gottwerdung in Alten Ägypten* (Munchen, 1977), the latter according to a book review by E. A. Reymond in *Bibliotheca Orientalis 37* (no. 5/6, Sep/Nov 1980), 313–315.
4. Hermann Kees, *Ancient Egypt: A Cultural Topography*, trans. by Ian F. D. Morrow, ed. by T. G. H. James (Chicago, 1961), 17, 47; Henri Frankfort, *et al., Before Philosophy: the Intellectual Adventure of Ancient Man* (Baltimore, 1949), 40; John A. Wilson wrote the chapters on Egypt. The Aswan High Dam now prevents most of the Nile's water from reaching the sea; see Robert P. Ambroggi, "Water," *Scientific American 243* (no. 3, September 1980): 101–116.
5. Miriam Lichtheim, *Ancient Egyptian Literature: a Book of Readings*. Vol. I: *The Old and Middle Kingdoms* (Berkeley, Calif., 1975), 196. One "instruction," probably an ethical teaching, has been attributed to Imhotep, but this

is not verifiable; see Sigfried Morenz, *Egyptian Religion*, trans. by Ann E. Keep (1960; English trans., Ithaca, N.Y., 1973), 111.

6. Wildung, *Saints* (n. 3), 31–32; Hurry, *Imhotep* (n. 3), 18–20; Kees, *Topography* (n. 4), 154; Morenz, *Egyptian Religion* (n. 5), 225; I. E. S. Edwards, *The Pyramids of Egypt*, rev. ed. (Harmondsworth, England, 1985), 278 (this book is probably the single best introduction to the pyramids).
7. Henri Frankfort, *The Birth of Civilization in the Near East* (1951; rprt. ed. New York, 1956), 99–100; Hurry, *Imhotep* (n. 3), 4–11; Gardiner, *Pharaohs* (n. 3), 72–76.
8. Hurry, *Imhotep* (n. 3), 3, 5; E. A. Wallis Budge, *The Egyptian Book of the Dead: The Papyrus of Ani* (1895; rprt. ed. New York, 1967), xlviii, cxxx, 89, 308.
9. Frankfort, *et al.*, *Before Philosophy* (n. 4), 95–96. Also see: Budge, *Book of the Dead* (n. 8), 69–81; Adolf Erman, *Life in Ancient Egypt*, H. M. Tirard, trans. (1894; rprt. ed., New York, 1971), 307–308; M. Zakaria Gonem, *The Lost Pyramid* (New York, 1956), 3–27; Morenz, *Egyptian Religion* (n. 5), 206. James H. Breasted, in *Development of Religion and Thought in Ancient Egypt* (1912; rprt. ed. Philadelphia, 1972), 52–55, emphasizes that the *ka* was a corporeal "superior genius intended to guide the fortunes of the individual *in the hereafter*," the *ka*'s chief habitat; it was the world's first "guardian angel."
10. Edwards, *Pyramids* (n. 6), 34–41.
11. W. Stevenson Smith, *The Art and Architecture of Ancient Egypt*, rev. by William Kelly Simpson (Harmondsworth, England, 1981), 42–43.
12. David O'Connor, "The Earliest Pharaohs and The University Museum," *Expedition 9* (1987): 27–39. Also see W. B. Emery, *Archaic Egypt* (1961; rprt. ed., Harmondsworth, England, 1987), 144–146. It has been suggested (Farouk El-Baz, "Desert Builders Knew a Good Thing When They Saw It," *Smithsonian 12* [1981]: 116–122) that perhaps ancient Egyptian builders, including Imhotep, modelled pyramids, and even the Sphinx at Giza, on natural rock forms, especially those showing distinctive patterns of erosion. Although this proposal does not exclude any of those outlined in the text, I would guess that the ancient builders' concepts were more likely to have been secondarily reinforced, rather than inspired, by the naturally shaped geological masses around them.
13. Edwards, *Pyramids* (n. 6), 41–55; R. Engelbach, "Mechanical and Technical Processes," in S. R. K. Glanville, ed., *The Legacy of Egypt* (Oxford, 1942), 120–159; Jean-Phillipe Lauer, *Les Pyramides de Sakkarah* (Cairo, 1977), 6–9; Aldred, *Egyptian Art* (n. 2), 51.
14. O'Connor, "Earliest Pharaohs," (n. 12).
15. Lauer, *Les Pyramides* (n. 13), 6–9. The only textual mention of Imhotep to have survived from his own lifetime is on the base of a statue of his king: "The seal-bearer of the King of Lower Egypt, . . . ruler of the great house, . . . the high priest of Heliopolis, Imhotep [is] the chief of sculptors, of the masons and of the producers of stone-vessels." (Wildung, *Saints* [no. 3], 31–32).

16. Edwards, *Pyramids* (n. 6), 41; Morenz, *Egyptian Religion* (n. 5), 203–204.
17. George Sarton, *A History of Science: Ancient Science Through the Golden Age of Greece* (Cambridge, Mass., 1952), 30.
18. Edwards, *Pyramids* (n. 6), 284–285; Baines and Málek, *Atlas* (n. 2), 140–141.
19. Gonem, *Lost Pyramid* (n. 9), 3–27, 167; Edwards, *Pyramids* (n. 6), 273–278; Breasted, *Religion* (n. 9), 71–74; Frankfort, *et al., Before Philosophy* (n. 4), 60; Aldred, *Egyptian Art* (n. 2), 47–48, 59–60.

CHAPTER ONE

1. Henry E. Sigerist, *A History of Medicine: Primitive and Archaic Medicine* (New York, 1951), 272, 323; Cyril Aldred, *Egyptian Art* (New York, 1980), 11–15; Ange-Pierre Leca, *La Médecine Égyptienne au Temps des Pharaons* (Paris, 1971), 167–378, *passim*.
2. Siegfried Morenz, *Egyptian Religion*, Ann E. Keep, trans. (1960; Engl. trans. Ithaca, N.Y., 1973), xii–xiv, 6–7, 11.
3. *Ibid.*, 42, 186–189, 192, 197–198.
4. Alan H. Gardiner, ed., *Hieratic Papyri in the British Museum, Ser. 3, Chester Beatty Gift*, I. *Text* (London, 1935), 50–51.
5. Miriam Lichtheim, *Ancient Egyptian Literature: A Book of Readings* Vol. III: *The Late Period* (Berkeley, Calif., 1980), 90–94. Also see: Paul Ghalioungui, *The Physicans of Pharaonic Egypt* (Cairo, 1983), 78–79. Although this compilation seems to be as complete as the available evidence allows, there are gaps in Ghalioungui's analyses (but none of the gaps substantially affects any of my own arguments); see Robert K. Ritner's book review in *Journal of Near Eastern Studies 47* (1988): 199–201.
6. F. Ll. Griffith and Herbert Thompson, eds., *The Leyden Papyrus: an Egyptian Magical Book* (publ. 1904 as *The Demotic Magical Papyrus of London and Leiden*; rprt. ed. New York, 1974), 125–129,
7. *Ibid.*, 95, 149–151, 187, 203.
8. B[endix] Ebbell, *The Papyrus Ebers: the Greatest Egyptian Medical Document* (Copenhagen, 1937), 29–30.
9. *Ibid.*, 30.
10. Paul Ghalioungui, *The House of Life: Magic and Medical Science in Ancient Egypt*, 2nd ed. (Amsterdam, 1973), 10; Leca, *Médecine* (n. 1), 69–73; Lydia Mez-Mangold, *A History of Drugs* (Basel, 1971), 25. For some representative amulets see: Edward Brovarski, Susan K. Doll, and Rita E. Freed, eds., *Egypt's Golden Age: the Art of Living in the New Kingdom, 1558–1085 B.C.* (Boston, 1982), 250–254.
11. Leca, *Médecine* (n. 1), 73–76, and Pl. 1; Claude Traunecker, "Une Chapelle de Magie Guérisseuse sur le Parvis du Temple de Mout à Karnak," *Journal of the American Research Center in Egypt 20* (1983): 65–92; Mohamed Saleh and Hourig Sourouzian, *Official Catalogue, The Egyptian Museum, Cairo* (Cairo, 1987), no. 261; Mez-Mangold, *Drugs* (n. 10), 18–19.

12. Francois Daumas, "Le Sanitorium de Dendara," *Bulletin de l'Institut Français d'Archéologie Orientale 56* (1957): 35–57. Examples of Egyptian incubations will be found in the Epilogue.
13. Ghalioungui, *Physicians* (n. 5), 11–12. Frans Jonckheere's *Les Médicins de l'Égypte Pharaonique: Essai de Prosopographie* (Brussels, 1958) was the first attempt to catalogue all the known Egyptian physicians, but Dr. Ghalioungui's is now the single most comprehensive collation of all the documentable pre-Ptolemaic physicians and physician-priests.
14. Ghalioungui, *Physicians* (n. 5), 9–11; Frédérique von Känel, *Les Prêtres-Ouâb de Sekhmet et les Conjurateurs de Serket* (Paris, 1984), 236, 278–279, 282–283, 302–305 (in which it is well argued that the medical skills of Sekhmet-priests were indistinguishable from those of the *swnw*).
15. Owsei Temkin, "Recent Publications on Egyptian and Babylonian Medicine," *Bulletin of the History of Medicine 4* (1936): 247–256.
16. Ghaloungui, *Physicians* (n. 5), 65.
17. Leca, *Médecine* (n. 1), 129–153; Ghalioungui, *Physicians* (n. 5), 89.
18. For a catalogue of the Egyptians' anatomic terms see: Gustave Lefebvre, "Tableau des Parties du Corps Humain Mentionnées par les Égyptiens," *Supplément aux Annales du Service des Antiquités 17* (1952). For the autopsies, see Ghalioungui, *Physicians* (n. 5), 7. A perhaps excessively harsh judgment is implicit in the discussion by P. M. Fraser, in *Ptolemaic Alexandria*, 3 vols. (Oxford, 1972), I, 344, of Egyptian civilization's "chronic inability to draw inferences and establish general principles from practical knowledge." However, he may not have been too far off the mark when it comes to medical topics.
19. Alan H. Gardiner, "The House of Life," *Journal of Egyptian Archaeology 24* (1938): 157–179; Labib Habachi and Paul Ghalioungui, "The 'House of Life' of Bubastis," *Chronique d'Égypte 46* (1971): 59–71; Lichtheim, *Literature* (n. 5), 36–41; Ghalioungui, *Physicians* (n. 5), 31–32, 66, 91–92; von Känel, *Les Prêtres-Ouâb* (n. 14), 379.
20. Vivian Nutton, "Museums and Medical Schools in Classical Antiquity," *History of Education 4* (1975): 3–15; Darrel W. Amundsen and Gary B. Ferngren, "The Forensic Role of Physicians in Ptolemaic and Roman Egypt," *Bulletin of the History of Medicine 52* (1978): 336–353; Fraser, *Alexandria* (n. 18), 338–344; Ghalioungui, *House of Life* (n. 10), 66.
21. Ghalioungui, *Physicians* (n. 5), 16–34, 38–50.
22. *Ibid.*, 43–44.
23. Herodotus, *The Histories*, Aubrey de Sélincourt, trans. (Baltimore, 1954), 132.
24. Ghalioungui, *Physicians* (n. 5), 44, 75; Robert O. Steuer, "*wḫdw*, Aetiological Principle of Pyaemia in Ancient Egyptian Medicine," *Bulletin of the History of Medicine Supplement No. 10* (1948), 10.
25. John Scarborough to J. Worth Estes, 22 August 1979. The translation cited by Ghalioungui (n. 5) on p. 44 may also follow Scarborough's thinking.

26. O. Kimball Armayor, "Did Herodotus Ever Go to Egypt?," *Journal of the American Research Center, Egypt 15* (1978): 59–73.
27. Ghalioungui, *Physicians* (n. 5), 43–44.
28. Paul Ghalioungui, "Did a Dental Profession Exist in Ancient Egypt?," *Medical History 15* (1971): 92–94; Ghalioungui, *Physicians* (n. 5), 43–45; Wendy Wood, "A Reconstruction of the Reliefs of Hesy-Re," *Journal of the American Research Center in Egypt 15* (1978): 9–24; Ebbell, *Papyrus Ebers* (n. 8), 103–104. A man found in a tomb at Kerma in the Sudan had had his upper central incisors extracted during adolescence, probably involuntarily, but he was probably not an Egyptian; Christian Simon, "Preliminary Anthropological Study of the Material from Kerma (Sudan): the 1984–1986 Campaign," *Genava*, n.s., *34* (1986): 29–33.
29. Ghalioungui, *Physicians* (n. 5), 18, 65, 92.
30. Frans Jonckheere, "Coup d'Oeil sur la Médecine Égyptienne: l'Intérêt des Documents non Médicaux," *Chronique d'Égypte 20* (1945): 24–32; Paul Ghalioungui, "Les Plus Anciennes Femmes-Médecins de l'Histoire," *Bulletin de l'Institut Français d'Archéologie Orientale 75* (1975): 159–164.
31. Ghalioungui, *Physicians* (n. 5), 73–74.
32. Louise Bradbury, "Nefer's Inscription: on the Death Date of Queen Ahmose-Nefertary and the Dead Found Pleasing to the King," *Journal of the American Research Center in Egypt 22* (1985): 73–95 (wherein the translation given there—and here—is attributed to I. E. S. Edwards, in *Journal of Egyptian Archaeology 51* [1956]: 16–28); also see Ghalioungui, *Physicians* (n. 5), 28, 73.
33. Ghalioungui, *Physicians* (n. 5), 29, 97; Leca, *Médecine* (n. 1), 124, 127.
34. Leca, *Médecine* (n. 1), 125 and Pl. 4.
35. T. G. H. James, *Pharaoh's People: Scenes from Life in Imperial Egypt* (London: 1984), 241–244; O. A. W. Dilke, *Mathematics and Measurement* (London, 1987), 24, 46.
36. Ghalioungui, *Physicians* (n. 5), 95–96; Leca, *Médecine* (n. 1), 125.
37. I am most grateful to Yvonne J. Markowitz of the Boston Museum of Fine Arts and to Dr. Cynthia Rose of Brandeis University, for making this translation for me, especially because we could not find one in the literature. The hieroglyphic publication of the text is in Sir Alan Gardiner, ed., *Ramesside Administrative Documents* (London, 1948), 47–48. The anonymous *swnw* is no. 112 in Ghalioungui's list in *Physicians* (n. 5), 30.
38. Jac. J. Janssen, *Commodity Prices from the Ramessid Period: an Economic Study of the Village of Necropolis Workmen at Thebes* (Leiden, 1975), 534; B. G. Trigger, et *al. Ancient Egypt: a Social History* (Cambridge, 1983), 228.
39. Ghalioungui, *Physicians* (n. 5), 96; Sigerist, *History* (n. 1), 323. Although there is no direct evidence that *swnw* were employed in the pharaohs' armies, the circumstantial evidence (especially that of the Smith Papyrus, for which see Chapter Three) is highly suggestive; this hypothesis is seconded by Prof. Alan R. Schulman of Queen's College, New York, in his 22 Apr 1988 letter to me.

40. Ghalioungui, *Physicians* (n. 5), 77.
41. *Ibid.*, 77.
42. *Ibid.*, 78.
43. *Ibid.*, 80–81; Herodotus, *Histories* (n. 23), 174, 229.

CHAPTER TWO

1. Pliny, *Natural History*, 10 vols., H. Rackham *et al.*, trans. (Cambridge, Mass., 1938–1962), II, 634.
2. Edward Brovarski, Susan K. Doll, and Rita E. Freed, eds., *Egypt's Golden Age: the Art of Living in the New Kingdom 1558–1085 B.C.* (Boston, 1982), 37; T. G. H. James, *Pharaoh's People: Scenes from Life in Imperial Egypt* (London: 1984), 112–113.
3. James, *Pharoah's People* (N. 2), 113–115.
4. J. Lawrence Angel, "Health as Crucial Factor in the Changes from Hunting to Developed Farming in the Eastern Mediterranean," in: *Paleopathology of the Origins of Agriculture* (New York, 1984), 51–73.
5. S. Boyd Eaton and Melvin Konner, "Paleolithic Nutrition: a Consideration of Its Nature and Current Implications," *New England Journal of Medicine 312* (1985): 283–289; letter, S. Boyd Eaton to J. Worth Estes, 17 Apr 1985, and accompanying photocopied typescript of "Selected Nutrient Values for Wild Game and Domestic Meat;" Henry E. Sigerist, *A History of Medicine.* Vol. I: *Primitive and Archaic Medicine* (New York, 1951), 249.
6. William J. Darby, Paul Ghalioungui, and Louis Grivetti, *Food: the Gift of Osiris*, 2 vols. (New York, 1977), I, 139–156, 172–189, 211–261, 265–318, 337–379, 396; II, 529–532, 552–579; H. M. Hecker, "A Zooarchaeological Inquiry into Pork Consumption in Egypt from Prehistoric to New Kingdom Times," *Journal of the American Research Center in Egypt 19* (1982): 59–71; Brovarski, *et al., Golden Age* (n. 2), 107–109. For the taboo fish, see Sue D'Auria, Peter Lacovara, and Catherine H. Roerig, eds., *Mummies and Magic: the Funerary Arts of Ancient Egypt* (Boston, 1988), 244.
7. D'Auria, *et al., Mummies and Magic* (n .6), 108–113; Darby, *et al., Food* (n. 6), I, 430–439, II, 461–486, 501–528.
8. Darby, *et al., Food* (n. 6), II, 653–753; L. Saffirio, "Food and Dietary Habits in Ancient Egypt," *Journal of Human Evolution 1* (1972): 297–305; Philip D. Curtin, "Nutrition in African History," *Journal of Interdisciplinary History 14* (1983): 371–382.
9. Darby, *et al., Food* (n. 6), II, 764–784, 791–807.
10. Saffirio, "Food habits" (n. 8); W. B. Emery, *Archaic Egypt* (1961; rprt. ed., Harmondsworth, England, 1987), 243–246; Naphtali Lewis, *Life in Egypt under Roman Rule* (Oxford, 1985), 69.
11. Sigerist, *History* (n. 5), 250; Mohamed Saleh and Hourig Sourouzian, *Official Catalogue, the Egyptian Museum, Cairo* (Cairo, 1987), nos. 140, 148, 231; W. Stevenson Smith, *The Art and Architecture of Ancient Egypt*, rev. by

William Kelly Simpson (Harmondsworth, England, 1981), 107, 213; Rita E. Freed, *Ramesses the Great* (Boston, 1988), 162, 164; Stephen P. Harvey, *Gifts to Osiris, Checklist of the Exhibition at the Yale University Art Gallery 18 February–3 May 1987* (New Haven, 1987), 12; the translation was transcribed from the exhibition label, while the entire stele is shown in the checklist.

12. Jacques Vandier, *La Famine dans 1'Égypte Ancienne* (Cairo, 1936), 1–4, 45–47; Freed, *Ramesses* (n. 11), 76. Many papers in the issue on "Hunger and History" of the *Journal of Interdisciplinary History 14* (1983), 199–534, clearly illustrate the multiple difficulties inherent in the assumption that famine inevitably leads to increased mortality. Still, for the moment I will agree that it is a reasonable first assumption, as argued in that special issue by Thomas McKeown in his paper "Food, Infection, and Population," 227–247.
13. Miriam Lichtheim, *Ancient Egyptian Literature: a Book of Readings*. Vol. III: *The Late Period* (Berkeley, Cal., 1980), 94–103; Vandier, *Famine* (n. 12), 41–42.
14. Étienne Drioton, "Une Représentation de la Famine sur un Bas-Relief Égyptien de la Ve Dynastie," *Bulletin de L'Institut d'Égypte 25* (1943): 45–54; Smith, *Art and Architecture* (n. 11), 133–134; Paul Ghalioungui, *The House of Life: Magic and Medical Science in Ancient Egypt* (Amsterdam, 1973), 154.
15. James, *Pharaoh's People* (n. 2), 114.
16. Karl W. Butzer, *Early Hydraulic Civilization in Egypt: a Study in Cultural Ecology* (Chicago, 1976), xiv, 6–9, 26–27, 59, 77–80.
17. *Ibid.*, 28–33, 51, 82–89; Barbara Bell, "The Dark Ages in Ancient History. I. The First Dark Age in Egypt," *American Journal of Archaeology 75* (1971): 1–26; Barbara Bell, "Climate and the History of Egypt: the Middle Kingdom," *ibid. 79* (1975): 223–269. In "Civilizations: Organisms or Systems?," *American Scientist 68* (1980): 517–523, Karl W. Butzer uses such data to support his view of "civilizations as ecosystems that emerge in response to sites of ecological opportunities, that is, econiches to be exploited." Thus, as the Egyptians opened more land to cultivation, they could feed more people at a constant food/person ratio. For data relating low Nile floods to climate, and presumably to crop production, see: Fekri A. Hassan, "Historical Nile Floods and Their Implications for Climactic Change," *Science 212* (1981): 1142–1145.
18. Hans Goedicke, *Lexikon der Ägyptologie* (Wiesbaden, 1984), V, 918–919; Francis L. Black, "Infectious Disease in Primitive Societies," *Science 187* (1975): 515–518; Robert M. May, "Parasitic Infections as Regulators of Animal Populations," *American Scientist 71* (1983): 36–45. However, as will be seen later, young Egyptians were susceptible to illnesses (probably infectious) that were severe enough to retard bone growth temporarily. A recent study I have not yet been able to examine is reported to have found little fluctuation in skeletal indicators of disease stress (see the growth arrest

lines discussed below) except during the First Intermediate and Late Periods, "suggesting consistent health patterns in Egypt broken only during periods of political instability;" see note by Robert Ritner, in *Newsletter 16* of the Society for Ancient Medicine and Pharmacy (1988), 46, in which he summarizes Jerilyn Pecotte's unpublished Ph.D. dissertation on *Temporal Trends in Biological Stress Indicators from Two Dynastic Egyptian Mortuary Samples*. (University of Utah, 1986).

19. See, for example, Thomas McKeown, *The Role of Medicine: Dream, Mirage, or Nemesis?*, 2nd ed. (Princeton, 1979).
20. Don E. Dumond, "The Limitation of Human Population: a Natural History," *Science 187* (1975): 713–721. Dumond postulates that before "modern history" began, mortality led to the loss of as many as 50 percent of all persons born before they could have reproduced, and that both fertility and mortality rates depended on available nutritional resources. In addition, a growing body of evidence suggests that women must have a critical mass of fat (which would be hard to maintain in the face of famine) to carry pregnancies successfully; Rose E. Frisch, "Fatness and Fertility," *Scientific American 258* (no. 3, March, 1988), 88–95.
21. J. Nemeskéri, "Some Comparisons of Egyptian and Early Eurasian Demographic Data," *Journal of Human Evolution 1* (1972): 171–186; Dumond, "Limitation" (n. 20).
22. M. Masali and B. Chiarelli, "Demographic Data on the Remains of Ancient Egyptians," *Journal of Human Evolution 1* (1972): 161–169. Women who bear children repeatedly after very short intervals do suffer energy drains that can, in turn, affect the health of their newborn infants; Frisch, "Fatness" (n. 20). Also see n. 19, Chapter Three.
23. Masali and Chiarelli, "Demographic Data" (n. 22).
24. Edward F. Wente, "Age of Death of Pharaohs of the New Kingdom, Determined from Historical Sources," in James E. Harris and Edward F. Wente, eds., *An X-Ray Atlas of the Royal Mummies* (Chicago, 1980), 234–285; Wilton Marion Krogman and Melvyn J. Baer, "Age at Death of Pharaohs of the New Kingdom, Determined by X-Ray Films," *ibid.*, 188–212.
25. Adolf Erman, *Life in Ancient Egypt*, H. M. Tirard, trans. (1886; rprt. trans. New York, 1971), 149, 408; Miriam Lichtheim, *Ancient Egyptian Literature*. Vol. II: *The New Kingdom* (Berkeley, Cal., 1976), 141; Ange-Pierre Leca, *La Médecine Égyptienne au Temps des Pharaons* (Paris, 1971), 409.
26. Leca, *Médecine* (n. 25), 405; Sigerist, *History* (n. 5), 222.
27. Sigerist, *History* (n. 5), 404, 419–420; Pliny, *Natural History* (n. 1), II, 483, 611–617; Frisch, "Fatness" (n. 20); Calvin Wells, *Bones, Bodies and Disease* (London, 1964), 180; McKeown, "Food" (n. 12).
28. Lichtheim, *Literature* (n. 25), 172; Leca, *Médecine* (n. 25), 411–424; Lewis, *Roman Rule* (n. 10), 219; Vern L. Bullough, *Sex, Society, and History* (New York, 1976), 37–42.
29. M. Masali, "Body Size and Proportion as Revealed by Bone Measurements

and their Meaning in Environmental Adaptation," *Journal of Human Evolution 1* (1972): 187–197; similar data are reported in: P. H. K. Gray, "The Radiography of Mummies of Ancient Egyptians," *ibid. 2* (1973): 51–53; and among the first measurements of ancient Egyptian bodies, Thomas Joseph Pettigrew, *A History of Egyptian Mummies* (London, 1834), 166–167. For growth rates, see George J. Armelagos, *et al.*, "Bone Growth and Development in Prehistoric Populations from Sudanese Nubia," *Journal of Human Evolution 1* (1972): 89–119. For the hardships of Egyptian farmers, see James, *Pharaoh's People* (n. 2), *passim*.

30. Leca, *Médecine* (n. 25), 420–421; Sir Marc Armand Ruffer, *Studies in the Palaeopathology of Egypt*, Roy L. Moodie, ed. (Chicago, 1919); A. C. Berry and R. J. Berry, "Origins and Relationships of the Ancient Egyptians. Based on a Study of Non-metrical Variations in the Skull," *Journal of Human Evolution 1* (1972): 199–208; D. L. Greene, "Dental Anthropology of Early Egypt and Nubia," *ibid.*, 315–324; R. C. Connolly, et al., "An Analysis of the Interrelationships between Pharaohs of the 18th Century," *MASCA* [Museum Applied Science Center for Archaeology, University of Pennsylvania, Philadelphia] *Journal 1* (1980): 178–181; Bernadine Z. Paulshock, "Tutankhamun and His Brothers," *Journal of the American Medical Association 244* (1980): 160–164.
31. The most recent large-scale study (of 160 specimens from three widely separated sites) is that of G. Paoli, "Further Biochemical and Immunological Investigations on Early Egyptian Remains," *Journal of Human Evolution 1* (1972): 457–466. He found incidences of 21.3 percent for blood group 0, 40.4 percent for group A, 21.3 percent for group B, and 17.5 percent for group AB (the incidences of each among modern American white subjects I have studied in my own laboratory were 37 percent 0, 39 percent A, 15 percent B, and 9 percent AB). Blood group typing with ancient bone material gives far different results (after subtracting the equivocal findings, 12.5 percent were of group 0, 7.5 percent A, 45.0 percent B, and 35 percent AB), according to S.M. Borgognini-Tarli and G. Paoli, "Biochemical and Immunological Investigations on Early Egyptian Remains," *ibid.*, 281–287
32. G. V. Hart, *et al.*, "Blood Group Testing of Ancient Materials," *MASCA Journal 1* (1980): 141–145; this paper is an excellent technical introduction to the subject.
33. Good modern descriptions of mummification, accompanied by those of ancient observers, such as Herodotus and Diodorus Siculus, are in: D'Auria, *et al., Mummies and Magic* (n. 6), 14–19, 71–72, 75, 111–112, and *passim*; Rosalie David, ed., *Mysteries of the Mummies* (London, 1978), 60–75; William H. Peck, "Mummies of Ancient Egypt," in Aidan Cockburn and Eve Cockburn, eds., *Mummies, Disease, and Ancient Cultures* (Cambridge, 1980), 11–28; Zaky Iskander, "Mummification in Ancient Egypt: Developments, History, and Techniques," in Harris and Wente, *X-Ray Atlas* (n. 24), 1–51; and Stuart Fleming, *et al., The Egyptian Mummy: Secrets and Science* (Phil-

adelphia, 1980). For a modern quasi-mummy, see Irving I. Lasky, "The Very Late Autopsy of Admiral John Paul Jones," *Forum on Medicine 3* (1980): 770–773.

34. A. B. Granville, *An Essay on Egyptian Mummies* (London, 1825), 8, 29–34.
35. Pettigrew, *History* (n. 29), 74, 155–168.
36. Warren R. Dawson and P. H. K. Gray, *Catalogue of Egyptian Antiquities in the British Museum*. Vol. I: *Mummies and Human Remains* (London, 1968), 30, 41–43.
37. Walter M. Whitehouse, "Radiologic Findings in the Royal Mummies," in Harris and Wente, *X-Ray Atlas* (n. 24), 286–297.
38. R. Ted Steinbock, *Paleopathological Diagnosis and Interpretation: Bone Disease in Ancient Human Populations* (Springfield, Ill., 1976), 171, 235, 264, 301–303, 322–324, 353–354, 389; I. Isherwood, H. Jarvis, and R. A. Fawcett, "Radiology of the Manchester Mummies," in A. Rosalie David, ed., *Manchester Museum Mummy Project. Multidisciplinary Research on Ancient Egyptian Mummified Remains* (Manchester, U.K., 1979), 25–64; P. H. K. Gray and Dorothy Slow, *Egyptian Mummies in the City of Liverpool Museums* (Liverpool, U.K., 1968); R. A. David, ed., *Science in Egyptology* (Manchester, U.K., 1986), *passim*; Fleming, *et al.*, *Egyptian Mummy* (n. 33), *passim*.
39. Typescript, "X-Rays of Mummies at the Museum of Fine Arts Photographed Jan. 16, 1933," 7 pp., no date, and unsigned typescript report, on stationery of Drs. Arial W. George and Ralph D. Leonard, October 24, 1940, 1 p., both in the Department of Egyptian and Ancient Near Eastern Art, Museum of Fine Arts, Boston; A. T. Sandison, "Diseases in Ancient Egypt," in Cockburn and Cockburn, *Mummies, Disease* (n. 33), 29–44.
40. Myron Marx and Sue Haney D'Auria, "CT Examination of Eleven Egyptian Mummies," *RadioGraphics* 6 (1986): 321–330; D'Auria, *et al.*, *Mummies and Magic* (n. 6), 105–106, 111–112, 169–171, 175, 207–208, 221, 246–247; Myron Marx and Sue H. D'Auria, "Three-Dimensional CT Reconstructions of an Ancient Human Egyptian Mummy," *American Journal of Roentgenology 150* (1988): 147–149.
41. W. M. Pahl, "Possibilities, Limitations and Prospects of Comuted Tomography as a Non-Invasive Method of Mummy Studies," in David, *Science* (n. 38), 13–24; F. P. Lisowski, "Prehistoric and Early Historic Trepanation," in Don Brothwell and A. T. Sandison, eds., *Diseases in Antiquity* (Springfield, Ill., 1967), 651–672.
42. Kent R. Weeks, "Ancient Egyptian Dentistry," in Harris and Wente, *X-Ray Atlas* (n. 24), 99–119; James E. Harris, Arthur T. Storey, and Paul V. Ponitz, "Dental Disease in the Royal Mummies," *ibid.*, 328–334; Dawson and Gray, *Catalogue* (n. 36), 42; Gray and Slow, *Egyptian Mummies* (n. 38), 69; F. F. Leek, "Dental Health and Disease in Ancient Egypt with Special Reference to the Manchester Mummies," in David, *Science* (n. 38), 35–42; N. J. D. Smith, "Dental Pathology in an Ancient Egyptian Population," *ibid.*, 43–48; F. F. Leek, "Cheops' Courtiers: their Skeletal Remains," ibid., 183

–199. Greene, "Dental Anthropology" (n. 30), notes caries in less than 1 percent of 397 remains in one series.

43. F. Filce Leek, "The Dental History of the Manchester Mummies," in David, *Manchester Museum* (n. 38), 65–77; R. Grilletto, "Caries and Dental Attrition in the Early Egyptians as Seen in the Turin Collections," in D. R. Brothwell and B. A. Chiarelli, eds., *Population Biology of the Ancient Egyptians* (London, 1973), 325–331.
44. James Henry Breasted, *The Edwin Smith Surgical Papyrus*, 2 vols. (Chicago, 1930), I, 303–305.
45. Weeks, "Egyptian Dentistry" (n. 42); Bernhard Wolf Weinberger, "The Dental Art in Ancient Egypt," *Journal of the American Dental Association 34* (1947): 170–184; James E. Harris and Paul V. Ponitz, "Dental Health in Ancient Egypt," in Cockburn and Cockburn, *Mummies, Disease* (n. 33), 45–51.
46. The discussion of collated autopsy findings in the next few paragraphs is based on many sources. Most have been succinctly summarized in Leca, *Médecine* (n. 25), *passim*. More recent findings are in: T. Aidan Cockburn, "Death and Disease in Ancient Egypt," *Science 181* (1973): 470–471, and amplified in *Paleopathology Newsletter* (Detroit), no. 1, March 1973; Fleming, *et al.*, *Egyptian Mummy* (n. 33); Cockburn and Cockburn, *Mummies, Disease* (n. 33); Aidan Cockburn and Eve Cockburn, "Autopsies in Mummies," *New England Journal of Medicine 305* (1981): 1534; a few others are scattered throughout David, *Science* (n. 38).
47. C. J. Hackett, "The Human Treponematoses," in Brothwell and Sandison, *Diseases* (n. 41), 152–169; Donald R. Hopkins, *Princes and Peasants: Smallpox in History* (Chicago, 1983), 14–16. If smallpox had been present in Egypt, I might have expected to find *some* documentary evidence of serious epidemic disease (even if the absence of such evidence cannot be assumed to imply that epidemics did not occur).
48. Sigerist, *History* (n. 5), 224.
49. Theodore E. Nash, *et al.*, "Schistosome Infections in Humans: Perspectives and Recent Findings," *Annals of Internal Medicine 97* (1982): 740–754; Halfdan Mahler, "People," *Scientific American 243* (September, 1980), 67–77; Robert P. Ambroggi, "Water," *ibid.*, 101–116.
50. Reinhard Hoeppli, "Hematuria Parasitaria and Urinary Calculi, Early Indications from Africa," *Acta Tropica 29* (1972): 205–217; P. B. Adamson, "Schistosomiasis in Antiquity," *Medical History 20* (1976): 176–188.
51. Chauncey D. Leake, *The Old Egyptian Medical Papyri* (Lawrence, Kans., 1952), 64, 91; Breasted, *Smith Papyrus* (n. 44), I, 472–487.
52. Aidan Cockburn, *et al.*, "Autopsy of an Egyptian Mummy," *Science 187* (1975): 1155–1160; Fleming, *et al.*, *Egyptian Mummy* (n. 33), 88–89; Hart, *et al.*, "Blood Group Testing," (n. 32).
53. S. W. Hillson, "Chronic Anaemias in the Nile Valley," *MASCA Journal 1* (1980), 172–174. Sigerist, writing 37 years ago, thought there was no evidence for malaria in ancient Egypt; *History* (n. 5), 224. However, immu-

nofluorescent-antibody testing and transmission electron microscopy have revealed evidence of malarial infection in the mummy of a 14-year-old boy who died around 1195 B.C.; Cockburn and Cockburn, "Autopsies" (n. 46).

54. Frederic Wood Jones, "The Post-Mortem Staining of Bone Produced by the Ante-Mortem Shedding of Blood," *British Medical Journal 1* (1908): 734–736.
55. Frederic Wood Jones, "The Examination of the Bodies of 100 Men Executed in Nubia in Roman Times," *ibid.*, 736–737.
56. O. V. Nielsen, P. Grandjean, and I. M. Shapiro, "Lead Retention in Ancient Nubian Bones, Teeth and Mummified Brains," in David, *Science* (n. 38), 25–33.
57. J. E. Wallgren, R. Caple, and A. C. Aufderheide, "Contributions of Nuclear Magnetic Resonance Studies to the Question of Alkaptonuria (Ochronosis) in an Egyptian Mummy," *ibid.*, 321–327.
58. E. Tapp and K. Wildsmith, "Endoscopy of Egyptian Mummies," *Ibid.*, 351–354.
59. A comprehensive overview with appropriate references to the literature is Paulshock's "Tutankhamun" (n. 30); follow-up letters to the editor include: David Kasanof, "Egyptian Artifacts," *Journal of the American Medical Association 244* (1980): 2730; Charles F. Timmons, "Genetics of the Eighteenth Dynasty," *ibid. 245* (1981): 1525; Bernadine Z. Paulshock, "Tutankhamun's Mother," *ibid. 249* (1983): 2178. For a "gallery" of portraits of Akhenaten, showing several versions of his body contours, see Saleh and Sourouzian, *Official Catalogue* (n. 11), nos. 159–166; the same volume also shows a fairly normal statue of Tutankhamun (no. 173). Some of the older arguments also appear in: Cyril Aldred and A. T. Sandison, "The Pharaoh Akhenaten: a Problem in Egyptology and Pathology," *Bulletin of the History of Medicine 36* (1962): 293–316; Egill Snorrason, "Cranial Deformation in the Reign of Akhaton," *ibid. 20* (1946): 601–610; Cyril Aldred, *Akhenaten, Pharaoh of Egypt—a New Study* (London, 1968), 133–139; Wells, *Bones* (n. 27), 108, 117; and Leca, *Médecine* (n. 25), 269.

CHAPTER THREE

1. The idea that surgeons focussed on "localized" conditions comes from Robert P. Hudson, *Disease and Its Control: the Shaping of Modern Thought* (New York, 1987), 66–67.
2. Frans Jonckheere, "Dans l'Arsenal Thérapeutique des Anciens Égyptiens," *Histoire de la Médecine 3* (1953): 9–24; René Fournier-Bégniez, "Médecine des Égyptiens," in: M. Laignel-Lavastine, ed., *Histoire Générale de la Médecine, de la Pharmacie, de l'Art Dentaire et de l'Art Vétérinaire*, 3 vols. (Paris, 1936), I, 89–128; Don Brothwell and A. T. Sandison, eds., *Diseases in Antiquity* (Springfield, Ill., 1967), *passim*; Henry E. Sigerist, *A History of Medicine*, Vol. I: *Primitive and Archaic Medicine* (New York and Oxford,

1951), 345; Sir Marc Armand Ruffer, *Studies in the Palaeopathology of Egypt*, Roy L. Moodie, ed. (Chicago, 1921), 200; Ange-Pierre Leca, *La Médecine Égyptienne au Temps des Pharaons* (Paris, 1971), 219, 433; Adolf Erman, *Life in Ancient Egypt*, trans. by H. M. Tirard (1894; rprt. ed. New York, 1971), 144; R. Ted Steinbock, *Paleopathological Diagnosis and Interpretation: Bone Diseases in Ancient Human Populations* (Springfield, Ill., 1976), 30–31, 37; T.G.H. James, *Pharaoh's People: Scenes from Life in Imperial Egypt* (London, 1984), 80, 92. The palpation of a possible hernia is in B. Ebbell, *The Papyrus Ebers: the Greatest Egyptian Medical Document* (Copenhagen, 1937), 123; "minor surgical procedures" are given on 120–128. Bilateral amputation appears to have been performed on a New Kingdom girl of about 13 years, perhaps because of a fall; E. Tapp, "The Unwrapping of 1770," in R.A. Davis, ed., *Science in Egyptology* (Manchester, England, 1986), 51–56.

3. James Henry Breasted, *The Edwin Smith Surgical Papyrus*, 2 vols. (Chicago, 1930), I, 365–366; Guido Majno, *The Healing Hand: Man and Wound in the Ancient World* (Cambridge, Mass., 1975), 89–90; Ebbell, *Papyrus Ebers* (n. 2), 125–127; Edward Brovarski, Susan K. Doll, and Rita E. Freed, eds., *Egypt's Golden Age: the Art of Living in the New Kingdom, 1558–1085 B.C.* (Boston, 1982), 57, 64. For a flint blade see: Sue D'Auria, Peter Lacovara, and Catherine H. Roehrig, eds., *Mummies and Magic: the Funerary Arts of Ancient Egypt* (Boston, 1988), 73.
4. Hermann Ranke, "Medicine and Surgery in Ancient Egypt," *Bulletin of the History of Medicine 1* (1933): 237–257; Jonckheere, "Arsenal Thérapeutique" (n. 2).
5. Alexandre Badawi, *Kom-Ombo Sanctuaries* (Cairo, n.d., but about 1920), 41. The ambiguous inscription reads: [Haoeris, one of the gods of the temple, is] "the true god who takes care of gods and goddesses. He with the two eyes, Lord of Ombos, the Great Hero who takes good care of him who loves him." The phrase "to take care of" need not imply only medical attention, of course.
6. Paul Ghalioungui, *The House of Life: Magic and Medical Science in Ancient Egypt*, 2nd ed. (Amsterdam, 1973), 100–102; Sigerist, *History* (n. 2), 345–346; Leca, *Médecine* (n. 2), 313; Ranke, "Medicine and Surgery" (n. 4).
7. For a comprehensive series of pictures of contemporary Greek and Roman instruments, see John Stuart Milne, *Surgical Instruments in Greek and Roman Times* (1907; rprt. ed. Chicago, 1976); for a small but very convincing selection of pictures, especially of speculums, see Lawrence J. Bliquez, "Greek and Roman Medicine," *Archaeology 34* (Mar/Apr 1981), no. 2: 11–17, and his "Roman Surgical Instruments in the Johns Hopkins University Institute of the History of Medicine," *Bulletin of the History of Medicine 56* (1982): 195–217. It has been argued that pan scales were not used for measuring drugs, but that inference seems unwarranted; see James, *Pharaoh's People* (n. 2), 256; Norman de G. Davies and R. O. Faulkner, "A Syrian Trading Venture to Egypt," *Journal of Egyptian Archaeology 33* (1947): 40

–46; and Brovarski, *et al., Golden Age* (n. 3), 58–60. Dr. Robert Bianchi of The Brooklyn Museum has been most helpful in providing information about tools such as those shown at Kom Ombo, although he does not think the instruments are for surgical use (letters to J. Worth Estes, 6 July 1981 and 16 July 1981). However, P. M. Fraser, in *Ptolemaic Alexandria*, 3 vols. (Oxford, 1972), II, 55, n. 321, says they are.

8. For possible examples of other nonmedical uses of at least some of the tools shown at Kom Ombo, see, e.g., Heinrich Schäfer and Walter Andrae, *Die Kunst des Alten Orients* (Berlin, 1942), 368, or the large plates in Norman de G. Davies, *The Tomb of the Two Sculptors at Thebes* (New York, 1925).
9. Paul Ghalioungui, "Did a Dental Profession Exist in Ancient Egypt?," *Medical History 15* (1971): 92–94; Bernhard Wolf Weinberger, "Did Dentistry Evolve from the Barbers, Blacksmiths, or from Medicine?," *Bulletin of the History of Medicine 8* (1940): 965–1011; Bernhard Wolf Weinberger, "Further Evidence that Dentistry was Practiced in Ancient Egypt, Phoenicia and Greece," *ibid. 20* (1946): 188–195; Bernhard Wolf Weinberger, "The Dental Art in Ancient Egypt," *Journal of the American Dental Association 34* (1947): 170–184. See Plate I at the end of Breasted, *Smith Papyrus* (n. 3) for one possible example of dental surgery.
10. F. Filce Leek, "Bite, Attrition and Associated Oral Conditions as Seen in Ancient Egyptian Skulls," *Journal of Human Evolution 1* (1972): 289–295; F. Filce Leek, "Teeth and Bread in Ancient Egypt," *Journal of Egyptian Archaeology 58* (1972): 126–132; D. L. Greene, "Dental Anthropology of Early Egypt and Nubia," *Journal of Human Evolution 1* (1972): 315–324; R. Grilletto, "Caries and Dental Attrition in the Early Egyptians as Seen in the Turin Collections," *Journal of Human Evolution 1* (1972): 325–331; Rosalie David, ed., *Mysteries of the Mummies* (London, 1978), 152; Merton Ian Satinoff, "The Medical Biology of the Early Egyptian Populations from Asswan, Assyut, and Gebelen," *Journal of Human Evolution 1* (1972): 247–257; George J. Armelagos, "Disease in Ancient Nubia," *Science 163* (1969): 255–259; Ghalioungui, *House of Life* (n. 6), 117; Aidan Cockburn, *et al.* "Autopsy of an Egyptian Mummy," *Science 187* (1975): 1155–1160; Leca, *Médecine* (n. 2), 307–316; Sigerist, *History* (n. 2), 346–349.
11. Ralph H. Major, *A History of Medicine*, 2 vols. (Springfield, Ill., 1954), I, 41; J. Bitschai and M. Leopold Brodny, *A History of Urology in Egypt* (1956), Fig. 2; Ebbell, *Papyrus Ebers* (n. 2), 103; Sigerist, *History* (n. 2), 244–248; Leca, *Médecine* (n. 2), 427; Ghalioungui, *House of Life* (n. 6), 93–98; Aidan and Eve Cockburn, eds., *Mummies, Disease, and Ancient Cultures* (Cambridge, 1980), 42; this volume includes detailed accounts of one Dynasty IV mummy who had been circumcised (18), and of three late mummies who had not (55, 77, 98). For examples of circumcised statues, see: Cyril Aldred, *Egypt to the End of the Old Kingdom* (New York, 1965), 124–125; Mohamed Saleh and Hourig Sourouzian, *Official Catalogue, the Egyptian Museum, Cairo* (Cairo, 1987), no. 64. An uncircumcised Dynasty IV youth of about ten years is shown in W. Stevenson Smith, *The Art and Architecture of*

Ancient Egypt, rev. by William Kelly Simpson (Harmondsworth, England, 1981), 139, and another from the Old Kingdom is in D'Auria, *et al.*, *Mummies and Magic* (n. 3), 89.

12. Alexander Badawy, *The Tomb of Nyhetep-Ptah at Giza and the Tomb of Ankhmahor at Saqqara* (Berkeley, Cal., 1978), 19; Maurice Pillet, "Les Scènes de Naissance et de Circoncision dans le Temple Nord-Est de Mout, à Karnak," *Annales du Service des Antiquities de l'Égypte 52* (1954): 77–104. James J. Walsh, in "First Pictures of Surgical Operations Extant," *Journal of the American Medical Association 49* (1907): 1593–1595, argues that the VI Dynasty relief may portray something other than simple circumcision, but no one seems to have agreed with him. Constant de Wit, in "La circoncision chez les anciens Égyptiens," *Zeitschrift fur Ägyptische Sprache 99* (1972): 41–48, postulates that circumcision was invented to relieve phimosis (a contraction of the foreskin that precludes its retraction), citing *Joshua 5*: 2–7, in which the Lord tells Joshua to "Make flint knives and circumcise the people of Israel again the second time," that is, those who have been born since they left Egypt; it was done at Gibeath-haaraloth, "the hill of foreskins," according to the Revised Standard Version. However, de Wit's train of thought connecting phimosis with *Joshua* is somewhat obscure to me. The honey ointment is mentioned in the Ebers Papyrus (Ebbell [n. 2], 103), but Ghalioungui (*House of Life* [n. 6], 89) argues that the Ebers recipe is really meant as an unguent for serious pricks by acacia thorns.
13. Dieter Müller, "Die Zeugung durch das Herz in Religion und Medizin der Ägypte," *Orientalia 35* (1966): 247–274; Calvin W. Schwabe, *Veterinary Medicine and Human Health*, 4th ed. (Baltimore, 1984), 255, 257; Ghalioungui, *House of Life* (n. 6), 111; H. Tristram Engelhardt, Jr., "The Disease of Masturbation: Values and Concept of Disease," *Bulletin of the History of Medicine 48* (1974): 234–248, esp. n. 39; Leca, *Médecine* (n. 2), 317–329; Oscar Sugar, "How the Sacrum Got Its Name," *Journal of the American Medical Association 257* (1987): 2061–2063. These connections are also clear in prayers to the gods, e.g., in Akhenaten's Great Hymn to the Aten and a later one to Khnum-Re, in which the god is said to have made "The loins to support the phallus / In the act of begetting." (Miriam Lichtheim, *Ancient Egyptian Literature*. Vol. II: *The New Kingdom* [Berkeley, Cal., 1976], 97; Vol. III: *The Late Period* [Berkeley, Cal., 1980], 111–113). The Greeks shared similar notions of parenthood: In Aeschylus's *Eumenides* (*The Oresteia*, trans. by Robert Fayles [Harmondsworth, 1977], 260), Apollo says, "The woman you call the mother of the child is not the parent, just a nurse to the seed. . . . The *man* is the source of life. . . . The father can father forth without a mother."
14. Serge Sauneron, "Les 'Dix Mois' Précédant la Naissance," *Bulletin de l'Institut Français Archéologique Orientale 58* (1959): 33–34; Darrel W. Amundsen and Gary B. Ferngren, "The Forensic Role of Physicians in Roman Law," *Bulletin of the History of Medicine 58* (1979): 39–56; Müller, "Die Zeugung" (n. 13); Ann Ellis Hanson, "The Eight Months' Child and the Etiquette of

Birth: *Obsit Omen!,*" *Bulletin of the History of Medicine 61* (1987): 589–602.

15. John M. Stevens, "Gynaecology from Ancient Egypt: the Papyrus Kahun: a Translation of the Oldest Treatise on Gynaecology that Has Survived from the Ancient World," *Medical Journal of Australia 2* (1975): 949–952. The original publication of this document was: F. Ll. Griffith, *Hieratic Papyri from Kahun and Gurob*, 2 vols. (London, 1898), 1, 5–11. Stevens' version is entirely compatible with Griffith's but more useful because the Victorian scholar felt compelled to translate all mentions of the female reproductive organs into Latin.
16. Stevens, "Gynaecology" (n. 15); Leca, *Médecine* (n. 2), 328; Ebbell, *Papyrus Ebers* (n. 2), 108.
17. P. Ghalioungui, Sh. Khalil, and A. R. Ammar, "On an Ancient Egyptian Method on Diagnosing Pregnancy and Determining Foetal Sex," *Medical History 7* (1963): 241–247.
18. Brovarski, *et al., Golden Age* (n. 3), 293–294; Leca, *Médecine* (n. 2), 298; Ebbell, *Papyrus Ebers* (n. 2), *passim*, for nonobstetric uses of human milk; also see MILK in the Appendix.
19. Ebbell, *Papyrus Ebers* (n. 2), 110, 113; Leca, *Médecine* (n. 2), 334–335; Stuart Fleming, *et al. The Egyptian Mummy: Secrets and Science* (Philadelphia, 1980), 60.
20. Ghalioungui, *House of Life* (n. 6), 114–116; Leca, *Médecine* (n. 2), 330–332; *Exodus 1*: 15–16 (Revised Standard Version); Pillet, "Scènes de Naissance" (n. 12); James, *Pharaoh's People* (n. 2), 227–228.
21. Stevens, "Gynaecology" (n. 15); Ebbell, *Papyrus Ebers* (n. 2), 108–113.
22. Breasted, *Smith Papyrus* (n. 3), gives the entire papyrus and a detailed translation in the first volume, while the second is a facsimile of the original hieratic script accompanied by its hieroglyph transliteration. A "consecutive translation," without editorial comment, is given in I, 429–466. Although Breasted's work is a major monument of modern scholarship in any field, some of his interpretations have since been modified or elaborated as exemplified in: Bruce Lawrence Ralston, "Medical Reinterpretation of Case Four of the Edwin Smith Surgical Papyrus," *Journal of Egyptian Archaeology 63* (1977): 116–121, and in Guenter B. Risse, "Rational Egyptian Surgery: a Cranial Injury Discussed in the *Edwin Smith Papyrus*," *Bulletin of the New York Academy of Medicine 48* (1972): 912–919; Ranke, "Medicine and Surgery" (n. 4); Henri Frankfort, *et al. Before Philosophy: the Intellectual Adventure of Ancient Man* (Baltimore, 1949), 105 (John A. Wilson wrote the section on Egypt).
23. Breasted, *Smith Papyrus* (n. 3), I, *passim*; George Sarton, "Book Review of Breasted, *The Edwin Smith Surgical Papyrus*," *Isis 15* (1931): 355–367; Risse, "Rational Egyptian Surgery" (n. 22); G. E. R. Lloyd, ed., *Hippocratic Writings*, J. Chadwick and W. N. Mann, *et al.*, trans. (Harmondsworth, England, 1978), 206. Also see n. 39 to Chapter One.

24. Majno, *Healing Hand* (n. 3), 84; P. H. K. Gray, "The Radiography of Mummies of Ancient Egyptians," *Journal of Human Evolution 2* (1973): 51–53; Leca, *Médecine* (n. 2), 370–373; Charles Bonnet, *Kerma: Territoire et Metropole* (Paris, 1986), 6, 46; Cyril B. Courville, "Injuries to the Skull and Brain in Ancient Egypt," *Bulletin of the Los Angeles Neurological Society 14* (1949): 53–85; John Baines and Jaromír Málek, *Atlas of Ancient Egypt* (New York, 1980), 203. Also see Plates II, VII, and VIII at the end of Breasted, *Smith Papyrus* (n. 3), for pictures of relevant battle wounds in mummies. If the Smith Papyrus was intended as a practical manual for treating soldiers and, perhaps, construction workers, it effectively contradicts the recent unsupported assertion that diseases of the lower class were "hardly considered at all and treatment for their complaints was minimal," made in P. B. Adamson's "Dracontiasis in Antiquity," *Medical History 32* (1988): 204–209. Many other documents cited in this book also refute Adamson's unwarranted assumption. Also see n. 7 to the Epilogue.
25. Breasted, *Smith Papyrus* (n. 3), I, 54–59, 217–224, 226–231, 363–369; Chauncey D. Leake, Sanford V. Larkey, and Henry F. Lutz, "The Management of Fractures According to the Hearst Medical Papyrus," in E. Ashworth Underwood, ed., *Science, Medicine, and History*, 2 vols. (London, 1953), I, 61–74; J. B. Bourke, "Trauma and Degenerative Disease in Ancient Egypt and Nubia," *Journal of Human Evolution 1* (1972): 225–232; G. Regöly-Mérei, "Surgery in Ancient Egypt," *Acta Chirurgica Academiae Scientiarum Hungaricae 13* (1974): 415–425; Satinoff, "Medical Biology" (n. 10); Ebbell, *Papyrus Ebers* (n. 2), 17; Majno, *Healing Hand* (n. 3), 92–95.
26. Breasted, *Smith Papyrus* (n. 3), 47–48, 134–135, and *passim*. Although Max Neuberger credited the Hippocratic authors with the first recognition of "spontaneous" healing ("An Historical Survey of the Concept of Nature from a Medical Viewpoint," *Isis 35* [1944]: 16–28), the same notion is surely implicit in the far older metaphor of the mooring stakes.
27. Breasted, *Smith Papyrus* (n. 3), 323–332. Hanging has long since been observed—and exploited—to cause erection; see, e.g., Richard J. Wolfe, "The Hang-up of Franz Kotzwara and Its Relationship to Sexual Quackery in Late Eighteenth-Century London," in: *Studies on Voltaire in the Eighteenth Century* (Oxford, 1984), 47–66.
28. Robert O. Steuer, "*wḫdw*, Aetiological Principle of Pyaemia in Ancient Egyptian Medicine," *Bulletin of the History of Medicine Supplement No. 10* (Baltimore, 1948), 19–20; Breasted, *Smith Papyrus* (n. 3), I, 57–59; Sarton, "Book Review" (n. 23); Majno, *Healing Hand* (n. 3), 97–107.
29. Erman, *Life* (n. 2), 468; Hermann Kees, *Ancient Egypt: a Cultural Topography*, ed. by T. G. H. James, trans. by Ian F. D. Morrow (Chicago, 1961), 117, 136; Pierre Montet, *Everyday Life in Egypt in the Days of Ramesses the Great*, A. R. Maxwell-Hyslop and Margaret S. Drower, trans. (1958; rprt. ed. Philadelphia, 1981), 142; Baines and Málek, *Atlas* (n. 24), 21; James Henry Breasted, *A History of Egypt*, 2nd ed. (1909; rprt. ed. New York,

1959), 112; Noel H. Gale and Zofia Stos-Gale, "Lead and Silver in the Ancient Aegean," *Scientific American 244*, no. 6 (June 1981), 176–192; Paul Raber, "Early Copper Production in the Polis Region, Western Cyprus," *Journal of Field Archaeology 14* (1987), 297–312. Other copper ores are mined today; see: Spencer R. Titley, "Porphyry Copper," *American Scientist 69* (1981): 632–638.

30. Ebbell, *Papyrus Ebers* (n. 2), 85 and *passim*; Stevens, "Gynaecology" (n. 15); Breasted, *Smith Papyrus* (n. 3).
31. Majno, *Healing Hand* (n. 3), 111–115.
32. These experiments, and those described below, were carried out in 1980–1981 by Stanley Strzempko, then a student at Colgate University working in my laboratory and now a resident in medicine. Similar results have since been obtained by graduate students in our department, according to their data as compiled for me by David Rosenbaum. Stevens, "Gynaecology" (n. 15); Anne E. Jones, "Folk Medicine in Living Memory in Wales," *Folk Life 14* (1976): 58–68. At least one biochemical explanation of copper's directly toxic effect on micro-organisms is demonstrated in: D. Bach, J. S. Britten, and M. Blank, "Polarographic Studies of Membrane Particles Containing Na-K ATPase," *Journal of Membrane Biology 11* (1973): 227–236.
33. Although myrrh has a long history of reported "antibacterial activity," such activity cannot be confirmed with modern assay methods; because myrrh must generally be dissolved in alcohol, perhaps its presumed antibacterial efficacy is attributable chiefly to the solvent. See, for instance: John Scarborough, "Nicander's Toxicology: Snakes," *Pharmacy in History 19* (1977): 3–23; T. E. Wallis, *Textbook of Pharmacognosy* (London, 1960), 492–495.
34. Ebell, *Papyrus Ebers* (n. 2), esp. 103 (for the circumcision ointment—but also see n. 12 above for a possible qualification) and 106 (for the ⅓ concentration); Chauncey D. Leake, *The Old Egyptian Medical Papyri* (Lawrence, Kans., 1952), *passim*; Frans Jonckheere, *Le Papyrus Médical Chester Beatty* (Bruxelles, 1947), 15–36; Breasted, *Smith Papyrus* (n. 3), *passim*.
35. Eva Crane, *The Archaeology of Beekeeping* (Ithaca, N.Y., 1983), 35–43.
36. Majno, *Healing Hand* (n. 3), 116–120; A. I. Root, *et al.*, *The ABC and XYZ of Bee Culture*, 4th ed. (Medina, Ohio, 1945), 535–538; Charles and C. P. Dadant, *Langstroth on the Hive and Honey Bee*, 23rd ed. (Hamilton, Ill., 1927), 405; Montet, *Everyday Life* (n. 29), 82; Nicholas Lemery, *Dictionnaire Universel des Drogues Simples*, ed. nouvelle (Paris, 1759), 713; Robert Blomfield, "Honey for Decubitus Ulcers," *Journal of the American Medical Association 224* (1973): 905; Nancy Condee, "Russian Remedies," *Wilson Quarterly*, summer 1988, 167–171.
37. It required an interpolated concentration of about 14 percent processed commercial honey to inhibit bacterial growth by 50 percent (a conventional measure of pharmacological effect), but a concentration of only 9 percent raw honey would accomplish the same end, whereas a concentration of 26 percent of the 80 percent glucose was required to achieve 50 percent in-

hibition. Thus, 80 percent glucose was only half as potent as the commercial honey, which in turn was only about two-thirds as potent as the raw honey.

CHAPTER FOUR

1. Ange-Pierre Leca, *La Médecine Égyptienne au Temps des Pharaons* (Paris, 1971), 403.
2. *Ibid.*, 233–242, 251–255, 279 (and Pl. IX), 291–296; Paul Ghalioungui, *The House of Life: Magic and Medical Science in Ancient Egypt*, 2nd ed. (Amsterdam, 1973), 86–88; J. Bitschai and M. Leopold Brodny, *A History of Urology in Egypt* (privately printed, 1956), *passim*.
3. W. Stevenson Smith, *The Art and Architecture of Ancient Egypt*, rev. by William Kelly Simpson (Harmondsworth, England, 1981), 345–346.
4. Mohamed Saleh and Hourig Sourouzian, *Official Catalogue, the Egyptian Museum, Cairo* (Cairo, 1987), no. 130; Paul Ghalioungui, "Sur Deux Formes d'Obésité Représentées dans l'Égypte Ancienne," *Annales du Service des Antiquitiés de l'Égypte 49* (1949): 303–316; Leca, *Médecine* (n. 1), 257–267, Pl. VIII; Cyril Aldred, *Egyptian Art in the Days of the Pharaohs, 3100–320 B.C.* (New York, 1980), figs. 30, 37, 71, 136, 137, 183.
5. Leca, *Médecine* (n. 1), 375, 467–468, and Pl. XV.
6. Sue D'Auria, Peter Lacovara, and Catherine H. Roehrig, eds., *Mummies and Magic: the Funerary Arts of Ancient Egypt* (Boston, 1988), 106–107; Frans Jonckheere, "Le Monde des Malades dans les Textes non Médicaux," *Chronique d'Égypte 25* (1950): 213–232; Frans Jonckheere, "Coup d'Oeil sur la Médecine Égyptienne: l'Intérêt des Documents non Médicaux," *Chronique d'Égypte 20* (1945): 24–32; A. Luca, "Poisons in Ancient Egypt," *Journal of Egyptian Archaelogy 24* (1938): 198–199; Henry E. Sigerist, *A History of Medicine*. Vol. I: *Primitive and Archaic Medicine* (New York, 1951), 334.
7. Jonckheere, "Coup d'Oeil" (n. 6); the hieratic inscription on an ostracon in the British Museum is given in *Inscriptions in the Hieratic and Demotic Character from the Collections of the British Museum* (London, 1868), Pls. XX–XXI, but no full translation seems to have been published, even if it has been cited frequently.
8. Miriam Lichtheim, *Ancient Egyptian Literature: A Book of Readings*. Vol. III: *The Late Period* (Berkeley, Calif., 1980), 18–19.
9. *Ibid.*, Vol. I: *The Old and Middle Kingdoms* (Berkeley, Calif., 1975), 61–63.
10. *Ibid.*, 163–169; the lines quoted are on 168.
11. Chris Thomas, "First Suicide Note?," *British Medical Journal 2* (1980): 284–285.
12. Lichtheim, *Literature* (n. 9), 163. Also see: Siegfried Morenz, *Egyptian Religion*, Ann E. Keep, trans. (1960; trans. ed. Ithaca, N.Y., 1973), 70–72, 183–213.

13. Dilip V. Jeste, *et al.*, "Did Schizophrenia Exist before the Eighteenth Century?," *Comprehensive Psychiatry* 26 (1985): 493–503.
14. Lichtheim, *Literature* (n. 8), 111–115; the lines quoted are on 112–113.
15. E. A. Wallis Budge, *The Book of the Dead: The Papyrus of Ani* (1895; rprt. ed. New York, 1967), 317; G. E. R. Lloyd, *Magic, Reason and Experience* (Cambridge, 1979), 231. Sir James George Frazer, *The Golden Bough: a Study in Magic and Religion* (abrgd., 1922; rprt. ed. New York, 1951), throughout provides many of the clues necessary for beginning to understand the ancient Egyptian's approaches to disease, although the book is relatively light on specifically Egyptian, much less medical, topics.
16. Robert O. Steuer and J. B. deC. M. Saunders, *Ancient Egyptian and Cnidian Medicine: the Relationship of Their Aetiological Concepts of Disease* (Berkeley, Calif., 1959), 1.
17. John A. Wilson, *The Culture of Ancient Egypt* (Chicago, 1951), 313; R. W. Sloley, "Science," in: S. R. K. Glanville, ed., *The Legacy of Egypt* (Oxford, 1942), 160–178.
18. Sigerist, *History* (n. 6), 349.
19. Henri Frankfort, *et al., Before Philosophy: the Intellectual Adventure of Ancient Man* (Baltimore, 1949), 66–68; Warren R. Dawson, *The Beginnings —Egypt and Assyria* (New York, 1930), 42–43; Morenz, *Religion* (n. 12), 126–130; Budge, *Book of the Dead* (n. 15), lxi, 189–212, 255, 293, 310–314; James H. Breasted, *Development of Religion and Thought in Ancient Egypt* (1912; rprt. ed. Philadelphia, 1972), 44, 55; D'Auria, *et al., Mummies and Magic* (n. 6), 30–31.
20. My summary of Egyptian pathophysiological concepts is based on the following publications. The most important documentary source is B. Ebbell, trans., *The Papyrus Ebers, the Greatest Egyptian Medical Document* (London and Copenhagen, 1937), 114–120. Its first major correlation with other Egyptian medical documents was that by James Henry Breasted, in *The Edwin Smith Surgical Papyrus*, 2 vols. (Chicago, 1930), I, 104–113. The final elucidation of the concepts of the *metu* and *wḫdw* emerged from the following series of studies: Robert O. Steuer, "*wḫdw*, Aetiological Principle of Pyaemia in Ancient Egyptian Medicine," *Bulletin of the History of Medicine Supplement No. 10* (Baltimore, 1948); Steuer and Saunders, *Egyptian and Cnidian Medicine* (n. 16); Robert O. Steuer, "Controversial Problems Concerning the Interpretation of the Physiological Treatises of *Papyrus Ebers*," *Isis 52* (1961): 372–380; and J.B. deC. M. Saunders, *The Transition from Ancient Egyptian to Greek Medicine* (Lawrence, Kans., 1963). Saunders and Steuer's interpretation of the direction of travel within the *metu* differs from older interpretations that assumed that *wḫdw* and all body fluids, including urine and feces, originated in the heart, but this probably seemed illogical even to the ancient physician. Also see Sigerist, *History* (n. 6), 349. The Egyptians were only the first to describe in writing a connection among air, breath, life, and the heart, a connection that has been perceived in virtually

all other cultures, for which see: Joachim S. Gravenstein, Santosh Kalhan, and Nikolas G. Balamoutsos, "Of Breath and Spirits," *Journal of the American Medical Association 246* (1981): 1091–1092.

21. Breasted, *Smith Papyrus* (n. 20), 111.
22. Guido Majno, *The Healing Hand: Man and Wound in the Ancient World* (Cambridge, Mass., 1975), 129; Sigerist, *History* (n. 6), 350–356; Ebbell, *Papyrus Ebers* (n. 20), 119–120.
23. Budge, *Book of the Dead* (n. 15), lviii–lix, 199–203; Breasted, *Religion* (n. 19), 301.
24. D'Auria *et al., Mummies and Magic* (n. 6), 228 (although I do not agree that medicine for the dead was necessarily equivalent to medicine for the living); Steuer and Saunders, *Egyptian and Cnidian Medicine* (n. 16), 3–4.
25. Steuer, "Aetiological Principle" (n. 20), 20. However, bleeding may possibly have been meant for treating a disease called *irwtn*, according to Chauncey D. Leake, *The Old Egyptian Medical Papyri* (Lawrence, Kans., 1952), 91.
26. Lichtheim, *Literature* (n. 8), III, 190.
27. Paul Ghalioungui, "La Notion de Maladie dans les Textes Égyptiens et ses Rapports avec la Théorie Humorale," *Bulletin de l'Institut Français d'Archéologie Orientale* 66 (1968): 37–48; Frankfort, *et al., Before Philosophy* (n. 19), 51; Budge, *Book of the Dead* (n. 15), 330–331; Owsei Temkin, *The Double Face of Janus* (Baltimore, 1977), 419–440.
28. "Seuche" entry in Hans Goedicke, *Lexikon der Ägyptologie* (Wiesbaden, 1984), V, 918–919; George Reisner, *The Hearst Medical Papyrus. Hieratic Text* (Leipzig, 1905), 5.
29. Breasted, *Smith Papyrus* (n. 20), 472–487.
30. Edward Brovarski, Susan K. Doll, and Rita E. Freed, eds., *Egypt's Golden Age: the Art of Living in the New Kingdom, 1558–1085 B.C.* (Boston, 1982), 31, 189–192, 199; Paul Honigsberg, "Sanitary Installations in Ancient Egypt," *Journal of the Egyptian Medical Association 23* (1940): 199–246; Rita E. Freed, *Ramesses the Great* (Boston, 1988), 181.
31. Steuer and Saunders, *Egyptian and Cnidian Medicine* (n. 16), 47, 53; T. G. H. James, *Pharaoh's People: Scenes from Life in Imperial Egypt* (London, 1984), 226–229; Honigsberg, "Sanitary Installations" (n. 30). For pictures of these latrines, see: J.E. Quibell, *Excavations at Saqqara (1912–1914). [Vol. 6] Archaic Mastabas* (Cairo, 1923), Pl. XXXI; J.D. Pendlebury, "Preliminary Report of Excavations at Tell El-Amarnah 1930-1," *Journal of Egyptian Archaeology 17* (1931): 233–244, Pls. LXX–LXXI; Seton Lloyd, "Model of a Tell El-Amarnah House," *ibid. 19* (1933): 1–7.
32. Herodotus, *The Histories*, trans. by Aubrey de Sélincourt (Baltimore, 1954), 131; Saunders, *Transition* (n. 20), 31. The Greek word *katharsis*, which can refer to laxative activity and to purification, may well have received both associations from the Greeks' more religiously oriented Egyptian neighbors. Indeed, the long testament of purity and preparedness in Chapter 125 of the *Book of the Dead* includes a promise that "my hinder parts are cleansed,"

which might well contain elements of both laxative activity and ritual purification (unless I, too, read too much between the lines); Budge, *Book of the Dead* (n. 15), 206–207.

33. Steuer, "Aetiological Principles" (n. 20), 10.
34. Leca's *Médecine* (n. 1), Ghalioungui's *House of Life* (n. 2), Breasted's *Smith Papyrus* (n. 20), Ebbell's *Papyrus Ebers* (n. 20), Chauncey D. Leake's *Medical Papyri* (Lawrence, Kans., 1952) (n. 25), and autopsy and X-ray data cited in Chapter Two, are the chief sources for most of the remainder of this chapter and will not be repeatedly cited unless there is a need to do so, although additional sources will be cited as appropriate.
35. Ghalioungui, *House of Life* (n. 2), 76–78; Breasted, *Smith Papyrus* (n. 20), 104, 109; Ebbell, *Papyrus Ebers* (n. 20), 114–115.
36. F. Daumas and P. Ghalioungui, "Quelques Représentations de Maladies Oculaires dans l'Ancienne Égypte," *Chronique d'Égypte 51* (1976): 17–29; Lise Manniche, "Symbolic Blindness," *Chronique d'Égypte 53* (1978): 13–21; Ch. L. Raemakers, "Un Symbole de la Chirurgie Oculaire Provenant de l'Ancienne Égypte," *Annales d'Oculistique 208* (1975): 161–166; Brovarski, *et al., Golden Age* (n. 30), 256; Arlington C. Krause, "Ancient Egyptian Ophthalmology," *Bulletin of the History of Medicine 1* (1933): 258–276; Leca, *Médecine* (n. 1), 283–306; Ghalioungui, *House of Life* (n. 2), 131; Ebbell, *Papyrus Ebers* (n. 20), 15. The English use of cataract derives from the analogy between the opacified lens and the obstruction to entering a castle imposed by a closed portcullis, according to the *Oxford English Dictionary*; the Latin *cataracta* means a waterfall, a portcullis, or a floodgate.
37. J. Worth Estes, "Dropsy," in Kenneth L. Kiple, ed., *Cambridge History and Geography of Disease* (in press).
38. Breasted, *Smith Papyrus* (n. 20), 104–109; Ebbell, *Papyrus Ebers* (n. 20), 115–116.
39. Ebbell, *Papyrus Ebers* (n. 20), 48; Leca, *Médecine* (n. 1), 173–181.
40. Dan Morse, Don R. Brothwell, and Peter J. Veko, "Tuberculosis in Ancient Egypt," *American Review of Respiratory Disease 90* (1964): 524–541; A. T. Sandison, "Evidence of Infective Disease," *Journal of Human Evolution 1* (1972): 213–224; Michael R. Zimmerman, "The Mummies from the Tomb of Nebwenenet: Paleopathology and Archeology," *Journal of the American Research Center in Egypt 14* (1977): 33–36; Frazer, *Golden Bough*, (n. 15), 422, 426, 442.
41. The problem here hinges on whether the number of papyric prescriptions reflects anything at all about disease incidence, real or only perceived. I suspect that the scarcity of antidiarrheal remedies in the papyri is analogous to the lack of fever remedies in the folk medicine of nineteenth-century isolated communities in the French Alps, a lack which has been interpreted to reflect resigned acceptance of diseases associated with fever in those peasant communities rather than freedom from such diseases, according to John Spears, in "Folk Medicine and Popular Attitudes toward Disease in the

High Alps, 1780–1870," *Bulletin of the History of Medicine 54* (1980): 303–336.

42. Leca, *Médecine* (n. 1), 197–200; Ghalioungui, *House of Life* (n. 2), 120–122; R. Ted Steinbock, *Paleopathological Diagnosis and Interpretation: Bone Diseases in Ancient Human Populations* (Springfield, Ill., 1976), 97.
43. Wilson, *Culture* (n. 17), 63, 78–79; Morenz, *Religion* (n. 12), 70–72, 183–213. However, during the decline of pharaonic power, in the last centuries B.C., Egyptians became less sure, and more skeptical, of their ability to overcome death. Thus, it may not be entirely coincidental that they acquired their first god of medicine at this time (see the Epilogue).

CHAPTER FIVE

1. Miriam Lichtheim, *Ancient Egyptian Literature*. Vol. III: *The Late Period* (Berkeley, Calif., 1980), 159–184, 200, 204.
2. The tablet, in the University of Pennsylvania Museum of Archaeology and Anthropology, Philadelphia, was translated by Michel Civil, in "Prescriptions Médicales Sumériennes," *Revue d'Assyriologie et d'Archéologie Orientale 54* (1960, no. 2): 59–72, and a summary is in Samuel Noah Kramer, "The World's Oldest Known Prescriptions," *Ciba Journal*, no. 12 (1959): 1–7 (both kindly supplied to me by the Museum). For the Sumerians' numbers see Jöran Friberg, "Numbers and Measures in the Earliest Written Records," *Scientific American 250* (no. 2, February, 1984), 110–118.
3. Henri Frankfort, *The Birth of Civilization in the Near East* (1951; rprt. ed. New York, 1956), 121–137; Civil, "Prescriptions" (n. 2).
4. Chauncey D. Leake, *The Old Egyptian Medical Papyri* (Lawrence, Kans., 1952), 89; G. Elliot Smith and Warren R. Dawson, *Egyptian Mummies* (London, 1924), 161–162; B. Ebbell, trans., *The Papyrus Ebers: the Greatest Egyptian Medical Document* (Copenhagen, 1937), 97, 106; Dioscorides, *The Greek Herbal*, trans. 1665 by John Goodyer, ed. by Robert T. Gunther (Oxford, 1934), 108; Warren R. Dawson, "The Mouse in Egyptian and Later Medicine," *Journal of Egyptian Archaeology 10* (1924): 83–86.
5. Frans Jonckheere, "Dans l'Arsenal Thérapeutique des Anciens Egyptiens," *Histoire de la Médecine 3* (1953): 9–24; Ange-Pierre Leca, *La Médecine Égyptienne au Temps des Pharaons* (Paris, 1971), 119; Henry E. Sigerist, *A History of Medicine*. Vol. I: *Primitive and Archaic Medicine* (New York, 1951), 343.
6. Edward Brovarski, Susan K. Doll, and Rita E. Freed, eds., *Egypt's Golden Age: the Art of Living in the New Kingdom, 1558–1085 B.C.* (Boston, 1982), 132.
7. Sir Alan Gardiner, *Egyptian Grammar*, 3rd ed. (Oxford, 1957), 197–199; Leake, *Medical Papyri* (n. 4), 20–25, 28–31.
8. Brovarski, *et al., Golden Age* (n. 6), 58–61. Karl M. Petruso, in "Early Weights and Weighing in Egypt and the Indus Valley," *Museum of Fine Arts*

(Boston) *Bulletin 79* (1981): 44–51, shows that the basic small weight used by the time of the New Kingdom was the *qedet*, or *kite* (one-tenth of a *deben*, for which see Chapter One), which weighed 9.1 grams.

9. Jonckheere, "Dans L'Arsenal" (n. 5).
10. Leake, *Medical Papyri* (n. 4), 28–33. For Egyptian mathematics see Richard J. Gillings, *Mathematics in the Time of the Pharaohs* (1972; rev. rprt. ed. New York 1982), esp. 210–213.
11. Ebbell, *Papyrus Ebers* (n. 4), 12.
12. Leake, *Medical Papyri* (n. 4), 50–51; George A. Reisner, *The Hearst Medical Papyrus. The Hieratic Text* (Leipzig, 1905), 4. Unfortunately, no complete consecutive English translation of the Hearst Papyrus has been published.
13. The original publication of the Kahun Papyrus was by F. Ll. Griffith, *Hieratic Papyri from Kahun and Gurob*, 2 vols. (London: 1898), I, 5–11. A more modern translation is by John M. Stevens, "Gynaecology from Ancient Egypt: the Papyrus Kahun, a Translation of the Oldest Treatise on Gynaecology that Has Survived from the Ancient World," *Medical Journal of Australia 2* (1975): 949–952 (see also n. 15 to Chapter Three).
14. Frans Jonckheere, *Le Papyrus Médical Chester Beatty* (Brussels, 1947), in which 15–36 are devoted solely to the translation (into French); the rest is commentary.
15. Frans Jonckheere, "Prescriptions médicales sur ostraca hiératiques," *Chronique d'Égypte 29* (1954): 46–61.
16. Leake, *Medical Papyri* (n. 4), 28–31; James Henry Breasted, *The Edwin Smith Papyrus*, 2 vols. (Chicago, 1930), I, 111–112.
17. Warren R. Dawson, "Studies in the Egyptian Medical Texts [III]," *Journal of Egyptian Archaeology 20* (1934): 41–46; Guido Majno, *The Healing Hand: Man and Wound in the Ancient World* (Cambridge, Mass., 1975), 109–111, 485; John C. Kramer, "Is *Djaret* the Ancient Egyptian Word for Opium?," unpublished MS., paper presented at annual meeting of the American Institute for the History of Pharmacy, 24 April 1979; Saber Gabra, "Papaver Species and Opium through the Ages," *Bulletin de l'Institut d'Égypte 37* (1956): 39–56; R. S. Merrillees, "Opium Trade in the Bronze Age Levant," *Antiquity 36* (1962): 287–292; R. S. Merrillees, *The Cypriote Bronze Age Pottery Found in Egypt* (Lund, Sweden, 1968), 154–161, and Pl. 36; Brovarski, *et al.*, *Golden Age* (n. 6), 59–60.
18. Ebbell, *Papyrus Ebers* (n. 4), 59–60.
19. A. Lucas, "Poisons in Ancient Egypt," *Journal of Egyptian Archaeology 24* (1938): 198–199; W.B. Emery, *Archaic Egypt* (1961; rprt. ed., Harmondsworth, England, 1987), 90; Charles Bonnet, "Archaeological Excavations at Kerma (Sudan)," *Genava*, n.s. *34* (1986): 5–20; Dale L. Morse, Laszlo Boros, and Peggy A. Findley, "More on Cyanide Poisoning from Laetrile," *New England Journal of Medicine 301* (1979): 892; Leca, *Médecine* (n. 5), 437–438; Leake, *Medical Papyri* (n. 4), 74–75.
20. Ebbell, *Papyrus Ebers* (n. 4), 70.

21. Sigerist, *History* (n. 5), 337, 341–343; Loren C. MacKinney, "Animal Substances in Materia Medica. A Study in the Persistence of the Primitive," *Journal of the History of Medicine and Allied Sciences 1* (1946): 149–170.
22. Paul Ghalioungui, *The House of Life: Magic and Medical Science in Ancient Egypt*, 2nd ed. (Amsterdam, 1973), 144–146; Christiane Desroches Nobelcourt, "Pots Anthropomorphes et Recettes Magico-Médicales dans l'Égypte Ancienne," *Revue d'Égyptologie* 9 (1952): 49–67; Sir James George Frazer, *The Golden Bough: a Study in Magic and Religion* (abrdgd. 1922; rprt. ed. New York, 1951), 12–52; G. E. R. Lloyd, *Magic, Reason and Experience* (Cambridge, 1979), 2.
23. Breasted, *Smith Papyrus* (n. 16), I, 2.
24. Owsei Temkin, "The Meaning of Medicine in Historical Perspective," in *The Double Face of Janus and Other Essays in the History of Medicine* (Baltimore, 1977), 41–49.
25. Leake, *Medical Papyri* (n. 4), 59, 81–84, 88, 95–96.
26. Sigerist, *History* (n. 5), 284.
27. Rita E. Freed, *Ramesses the Great, an Exhibition at the Boston Museum of Science* (Memphis, Tenn., 1987), 171; Brovarski, *et al., Golden Age* (n. 6), 97–100.
28. Lofty Boulos, *Medicinal Plants of North Africa* (Algonac, Mich., 1983); Thomas E. Keys, *The History of Surgical Anesthesia* (1945; rprt. ed., Huntington, N.Y., 1978), 5–11; Dioscorides, *Greek Herbal* (n. 4), 472–474; *Genesis* 30:14–16 (although it is not clear from this alone that the mandrake was actually used by Rachel as an aphrodisiac); Julius A. Brewer, *The Literature of the Old Testament* (rev. ed., New York, 1933), 75.
29. Walter H. Lewis and Memory P. P. Elvin-Lewis, *Medical Botany* (New York, 1977), 427.
30. This possibility emerges from my studies of patients' responses to eighteenth-century remedies, few of which were any more therapeutically selective than those of the *swnw*. See, e.g., J. Worth Estes, "Therapeutic Practice in Colonial New England," in: Philip Cash, Eric H. Christianson, and J. Worth Estes, eds., *Medicine in Colonial Massachusetts, 1620–1820* (Boston, 1980), 289–383, esp. 352–359; J. Worth Estes, "Naval Medicine in the Age of Sail: the Voyage of the *New York*, 1802–1803," *Bulletin of the History of Medicine* 56 (1982): 238–253; J. Worth Estes, "Drug Usage at the Infirmary: the Example of Dr. Andrew Duncan, Sr.," Appendix D in: Guenter B. Risse, *Hospital Life in Enlightenment Scotland: Care and Teaching at the Royal Infirmary of Edinburgh* (Cambridge, 1986), 351–384, esp. 365; also see 226–239 of Risse's text. "Cure rates" at the Edinburgh Infirmary were lower than those for the nearly contemporary American patient populations described in the first two papers cited above, for several good reasons, but, taken together, these data show that the vast majority of adult patients recovered after (or despite) their physicians' treatments. It would seem reasonable to infer that Egyptian patients fared about equally well at the hands

of the *swnw*, whose drugs were no "better" or "worse" than those of Western physicians in the eighteenth century.

31. Dioscorides, *Greek Herbal* (n. 4), 60. No new English translation has appeared since this 1655 version.
32. Geoffrey Keynes, ed., *The Works of Sir Thomas Browne*, 6 vols. (London, 1929), IV, 47–48 (from *Hydriotaphia: Urne-Buriall*); V, 459–463 (from "A Fragment on Mummies," although Keynes thought that Browne may not have written it himself).
33. *The Edinburgh New Dispensatory*, 4th ed. (Edinburgh, 1794), 576.
34. J. Worth Estes and LaVerne Kuhnke, "French Observations of Disease and Drug Use in Late Eighteenth-Century Cairo," *Journal of the History of Medicine & Allied Sciences 39* (1984): 121–152.
35. Reisner, *Hearst Medical Papyrus* (n. 12), 5.
36. Jonathan Cott, *The Search for Omm Sety* (New York, 1987), 93–99. Unfortunately, when we talked with Eady at Abydos in 1979, I had no idea I would undertake this book, nor that she could have told me about local folk medicine.
37. What follows is extracted from the typescript "An Interview with Hussein Mustapha Ahmed, self-styled *feki* of Karima, Sudan, March 15, 1987, by Timothy Kendall, with Cynthia Shartzer translating from Arabic," which Dr. Kendall gave me. I am most grateful to him for permission to include this extraordinary material here.
38. Ghada Karmi, "The Colonisation of Arabic Medicine," in Roy Porter, ed., *Patients and Practitioners: Lay Perceptions of Medicine in Pre-Industrial Society* (Cambridge, 1985), 315–339.

EPILOGUES

1. James Henry Breasted, *The Edwin Smith Surgical Papyrus*, 2 vols. (Chicago, 1930), I, xiii; George Sarton, book review of Breasted, *The Edwin Smith Surgical Papyrus, Isis 25* (1931): 355–367; Chauncey D. Leake, *The Old Egyptian Medical Papyri* (Lawrence, Kans., 1952), 16–17; Warren R. Dawson, *The Beginnings—Egypt and Assyria* (New York, 1930), *passim*; Henri Frankfort, *The Birth of Civilization in the Near East* (1951; rprt. ed. New York, 1956), 121–137.
2. John A. Wilson, *The Culture of Ancient Egypt* (Chicago, 1951), 313.
3. R. W. Sloley, "Science," in S. R. K. Glanville, ed., *The Legacy of Egypt* (Oxford, 1942), 160.
4. Warren R. Dawson, "Egypt's Place in Medical History," in: E. Ashworth Underwood, ed., *Science, Medicine, and History*, 2 vols. (London, 1953), I, 47–60, 48.
5. George Sarton, *A History of Science: Ancient Science Through the Golden Age of Greece* (Cambridge, Mass., 1952), 4, 48–49.
6. Sarton, review of *Smith Papyrus* (n. 1); Owsei Temkin, "Recent Publications

on Egyptian and Babylonian Medicine," *Bulletin of the History of Medicine 4* (1936): 247–256; Hermann Ranke, "Medicine and Surgery in Ancient Egypt," *Bulletin of the History of Medicine 1* (1933): 237–257.

7. Also see n. 30 to Chapter Five. Another supplementary explanation of why some dwellers on the Nile may have recovered from some infections has been proposed. Bones from a Nubian cemetery of 350–550 A.D. have provided possible evidence of regular ingestion of tetracycline antibiotics, perhaps produced fortuitously by *Streptomyces* fungi that might have contaminated the Nubians' grain stores. The evidence is not as complete as the investigators wished, but their argument is at least circumstantially compelling. However, while the tetracyclines are effective against a wide range of micro-organisms, it is certainly premature to conclude that the results of this serendipitous discovery "explain the extremely low rates of infectious disease found among" these early Christian Nubians. Everett J. Bassett, *et al.* "Tetracycline-Labeled Human Bone from Ancient Sudanese Nubia (A.D. 350)," *Science 209* (1980): 1532–1534.
8. John Boardman, *The Greeks Overseas*, 3rd ed. (London, 1980), 111–151.
9. Sarton, *History* (n. 5), 44; Sloley, "Science" (n. 3), 160.
10. Homer, *The Odyssey*, trans. by E. V. Rieu (Harmondsworth, England, 1946), 70 (Book IV).
11. James H. Breasted, *Development of Religion and Thought in Ancient Egypt* (1912; rprt. ed. Philadelphia, 1972), 368. A similar version of Egypt's reputation for her native medicines is found in *Jeremiah 46*: 11, where it is pointed out that "In vain you [i.e., the Egyptians] have used many medicines," because of their defeat by Nebuchadrezzar, king of Babylon, in 605 B.C. (R.S.V.).
12. A.S. Yahuda, "Medical and Anatomical Terms in the Pentateuch in the Light of Egyptian Medical Papyri," *Journal of the History of Medicine 2* (1947): 549–574.
13. Peter Brain, *Galen on Bloodletting* (Cambridge, 1986), 5, 11, 124.
14. Robert O. Steuer and J. B. deC. M. Saunders, *Ancient Egyptian and Cnidian Medicine: the Relationship of their Aetiological Concepts of Disease* (Berkeley, Cal., 1959), *passim*; J. B. deC. M. Saunders, *The Transitions from Ancient Egyptian to Greek Medicine* (Lawrence, Kans., 1963), *passim*; Steven M. Oberhelman, "The Diagnostic Dream in Ancient Medical Theory and Practice," *Bulletin of the History of Medicine 61* (1987): 47–60; Breasted, *Smith Papyrus* (n. 1), 476–477; Warren R. Dawson, *A Leechbook or Collection of Medical Recipes of the Fifteenth Century* (London, 1934), 12, 15. Not all scholars agree about the magnitude of Greece's medical debt to Egypt, or even if there was *any* such debt. Lloyd, for instance, has questioned the relative contributions of the diffusion of Egyptian medical knowledge to Greece and of its independent development in the two cultures; G. E. R. Lloyd, *Magic, Reason and Experience* (Cambridge, 1979), 10–29, 232, n. 21. P. M. Fraser goes so far as to postulate that Egyptian medical practices

influenced those taught at Alexandria only minimally; *Ptolemaic Alexandria*, 3 vols. (Oxford, 1972), I, 374–375, II, 498, n. 20. Several Egyptian plant remedies are still used in Greek folk medicine; Georges Sfikas, *Plantes Médicinales de la Grèce* (Athens, 1981), *passim*.

15. Max Neuberger, "An Historical Survey of the Concept of Nature from a Medical Viewpoint," *Isis 35* (1944): 16–28.
16. Paul Ghalioungui, "Ancient Egyptian Remedies and Medieval Arabic Writers," *Bulletin de l'Institut Français d'Archéologie Orientale 68* (1969): 41–51; Martin Levey, trans., *The Medical Formulary or Aqrābādhīn of Al-Kindī* (Madison, Wisc., 1966), *passim*, but see esp. 21; Michael W. Dols, *Medieval Islamic Medicine: Ibn Ridwan's Treatise "On the Prevention of Bodily Ills in Egypt"* (Berkeley, Calif., 1984), 12–13.
17. J. Worth Estes, "Therapeutic Practice in Colonial New England," in Philip Cash, Eric H. Christianson, and J. Worth Estes, eds., *Medicine in Colonial Massachusetts, 1620–1820* (Boston, 1980), 289–383; J. Worth Estes and LaVerne Kuhnke, "French Observations of Disease and Drug Use in Late Eighteenth-Century Cairo," *Journal of the History of Medicine and Allied Sciences 39* (1984): 121–152. Also see the Postscripts to Chapter Five.
18. Dietrich Wildung, *Egyptian Saints: Deification in Pharaonic Egypt* (New York, 1977), 75–77.
19. John Perkins, "Memoranda Medica," unpublished MS, Boston Medical Library, B.MSb64.0, 31.
20. Jamieson B. Hurry, *Imhotep: the Vizier and Physician of King Zoser*, 2nd ed. (London, 1928), 67; Sir Alan Gardiner, *Egypt of the Pharoahs* (London, 1961), 433.
21. Wildung, *Saints* (n. 18), 34; Hurry, *Imhotep* (n. 20), 56, 69; E. A. E. Reymond, review of Dietrich Wildung, *Imhotep und Amenhotep. Gottwerdung in Alten Ägypten* (Munchen, 1977), in: *Bibliotheca Orientalis 37* (no. 5/6, Sep/Nov 1980), 313–315; Cyril Aldred, *Egyptian Art* (New York, 1980), 150; Bernard P. Grenfell and Arthur S. Hunt, eds., *The Oxyrhynchus Papyrus. Part XI* (London, 1915), 221. For an account of another ancient Egyptian intellectual who was deified, see Wildung's *Saints*, 83–110; he was Amenhotep, Son-of-Hapu, who served his king, Amenhotep III (1391–1353 B.C.), in many of the capacities in which Zoser had employed Imhotep some thirteen centuries earlier.
22. Grenfell and Hunt, *Oxyrhynchus Papyrus* (n. 21), 230–231.
23. Hurry, *Imhotep* (n. 20), 65; Wildung, *Saints* (n. 18), 33, 38; Gardiner, *Egypt* (n. 20), 409, 433; James Henry Breasted, *A History of Egypt*, 2nd ed. (1909; rprt. ed. New York, 1959), 41–42; Aldred, *Egyptian Art* (n. 21), 45. Manetho also noted that the second pharoah of the First Dynasty, Athothis (also known as Hor-aḥa), "built the palace at Memphis; his anatomical works are extant, for he was a physician" (see Gardiner, *Egypt* [n. 20], 430). Manetho or his informants may have confused early legends that might also have included Imhotep and his king, or, more likely, Manetho may have confused Athothis

with Thoth; see, Thomas Greenhill, *ΝΕΚΡΟΚΗΔΕΙΑ: or, the Art of Embalming* (London, 1705), 170.

24. Wildung, *Saints* (n. 18), 43; Hurry, *Imhotep* (n. 20), 56–63; Grenfell and Hunt, *Oxyrhynchus Papyrus* (n. 21), 221–223; Aldred, *Egyptian Art* (n. 21), 228. The myths of Asklepios are recapitulated in: Robert Graves, *The Greek Myths*, 2 vols. in one (New York, 1957), I, 173–176. Associations between Imhotep and Asklepios are implicit, at least, in the cure of barrenness by the priests of Asklepios, in the provision of remedies through dreams (I, 178–179), in Asklepios' revival of Heracles after the hero had been murdered by Typhon (or Thon), the Greek form of Seth (II, 152), and in the dream episode recounted earlier (see n. 22).
25. Vern L. Bullough, *The Development of Medicine as a Profession* (New York, 1966), 1, 10–11; Sue D'Auria, Peter Lacovara, and Catherine H. Roehrig, eds., *Mummies and Magic: the Funerary Arts of Ancient Egypt* (Boston, 1988), 232.
26. Adolf Erman, *Life in Ancient Egypt*, trans. by H. M. Tirard (1894; rprt. ed. New York, 1971), 112.
27. Florence Nightingale, *Letters from Egypt. A Journey on the Nile, 1849–1850*, Anthony Sattin, ed. (New York, 1987), 161.
28. Erman, *Life* (n. 26), 273, 293; Hermann Kees, *Ancient Egypt: A Cultural Topography*, trans. by Ian F. D. Morrow, ed. by T. G. H. James (Chicago, 1961), 57–59, 68, 274, 281–283; Aldred, *Egyptian Art* (n. 21), 202; Henri Frankfort, *et al.*, *Before Philosophy: the Intellectual Adventure of Ancient Man* (Baltimore, 1949), 123–124.
29. T. G. H. James, *Pharaoh's People: Scenes from Life in Imperial Egypt* (London, 1984), 132–153.
30. Miriam Lichtheim, *Ancient Egyptian Literature*. Vol. II: *The New Kingdom* (Berkeley, Calif., 1976), 169.
31. Ibid., Vol. I: *The Old and Middle Kingdoms* (1975), 184–192.
32. Lichtheim, *Literature* (n. 30), 176–177.
33. Erman, *Life* (n. 26), 550.
34. Hurry, *Imhotep* (n. 20), 63–64; Wildung, *Saints* (n. 18), 43–47; Richard Lepzius, *Denkmaler aus Ägypten und Äthiopien* (Berlin, 1849–50), IX, Abt. 4, Pl. 18.
35. Hurry, *Imhotep* (n. 20), 16, 77–80, 103–104, 130–131; Wildung, *Saints* (n. 18), 66; Siegfried Morenz, *Egyptian Religion*, trans. by Ann E. Keep (1960; English trans. Ithaca, N.Y., 1973), 85.
36. Hurry, *Imhotep* (n. 20), 65–66; Wildung, *Saints* (n. 18), 50; Kees, *Topography* (n. 28), 161. Sir James Frazer, *The Golden Bough: a Study in Magic and Religion* (abrgd. 1922; rprt. ed. New York, 1951), 76–77, notes that, in many cultures, twins have been held to be especially magical, sometimes in relation to health; although I have no idea how twins were regarded late in Egyptian history, the appointment of twin sisters as Imhotep's priestesses cannot be devoid of all symbolism or magical import; and, according to

Graves, *Greek Myths* (n. 24), I, 1977, Asklepios had a twin. By Hurry's computations, Imhotep's birth would be commemorated today on 31 May, his death on 1 July, and his apotheosis on 19 April.

37. P. M. Fraser, *Alexandria* (n. 14), I, 375.
38. J. Grafton Milne, "The Sanatorium of Dêr-el-Bahri," *Journal of Egyptian Archaeology 1* (1914): 96–98; Wildung, *Saints* (n. 18), 63, 70; Hurry, *Imhotep* (n. 20), 49–55, 92–103. Both Hurry and Wildung list all the known sites associated with Imhotep that can still be seen in Egypt, but Hurry's directions for finding specific inscriptions are better (although he omits the inscription described in the next paragraph).
39. Lichtheim, *Literature* (n. 30), Vol. III: *The Late Period* (1980), (n. 30), 59–65.
40. *Ibid.*, 104–107.
41. Wildung, *Deification* (n. 18), 55; Morenz, *Egyptian Religion* (n. 35), 250, refers to Imhotep as "the Egyptian saviour hero," but this conclusion might well apply to other gods in the Egyptian pantheon. I am not even convinced that the phrase would be any more appropriate if it read "*an* Egyptian saviour hero."
42. Aldred, *Egyptian Art* (n. 21), 105.
43. Jacob Bigelow, *A History of the Cemetery of Mount Auburn* (Boston & Cambridge, 1860); Jacob Bigelow, "Remarks at Dedication of the Sphinx," 1872, MSS. B.MS C25.2, Boston Medical Library; *The Picturesque Pocket Companion, and Visitor's Guide, through Mount Auburn* (Boston, 1839); Barbara Rotundo, "Mount Auburn Cemetery: a Proper Boston Institution," *Harvard Library Bulletin 22* (1974): 268–279. For Bigelow's most important contribution to American medicine, see Richard J. Wolfe, *Jacob Bigelow's American Medical Botany 1817–1821* (North Hills, Penna., and Boston, 1979).

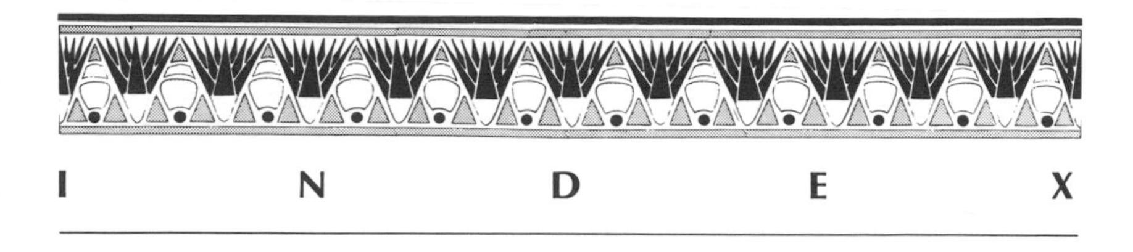

INDEX

All drug ingredients known or thought to have been used in ancient Egypt are listed alphabetically in the Appendix (pp. 136–157); additional mentions of some of those ingredients in the text are given below.